DID YOU KNOW?

* Heavy starch eaters are more susceptible to sinus and respirary infections. . . .

* A meal should be predominantly protein or carbohydrate, but never both. . . .

* Milk is fine for children, but of doubtful value to adults. . . .

* Spinach is one vegetable that is *not* recommended. . . .

* Honey is one of nature's most powerful germ killers. . . .

* A nervous system that is starved for protein and fat has no choice but to become jittery. . . .

LELORD KORDEL, world-famous nutritionist, explains how the food you eat can keep your body healthy, strong and youthful.

EAT AND GROW YOUNGER

LELORD KORDEL

MANOR BOOKS INC.

A MANOR BOOK......1976

Manor Books, Inc.
432 Park Avenue South
New York, New York 10016

Library of Congress Catalogue Card Number:
52-5176

CONTENTS

PART II: YOUR EAT-AND-GROW-YOUNGER DIET PROGRAM

EAT AND GROW YOUNGER

Part I: HOW TO STAY YOUNG

Chapter 1

OF COURSE YOU WANT TO STAY YOUNG!

Mr. U awoke one morning to a disturbing discovery. A panicky feeling welled up from the depths of the little pot-belly that had begun to bulge out below his belt.

He glanced across the breakfast table at Mrs. U.

Dismayed, he realized for the first time that the woman facing him was in the same unpleasant fix he now found himself:

He was getting old—and so was she!

Pushing aside his bowl of starchy cereal (liberally sprinkled with refined sugar), he laid down his slice of so-called "enriched" white bread toast. His usual zest for breakfast was gone.

Why did people have to grow old so soon? He was only forty-six. Why shouldn't he feel peppy and look young for at least another forty or fifty years?

Look at old Joe Jenks, who had lived on a neighboring farm when he was a boy.

Joe had gotten up before sunrise every morning, did more work than the hired man, ate heartily, slept like a top, took a young second wife, and pooh-poohed anybody who tried to tell him that his eighty-odd years made him a ready candidate for a coffin.

The old fellow had fooled the whole community by living, hale and hearty, well into his nineties.

What was wrong? Why shouldn't men and women keep on looking and feeling *young and alive* past that momentous fortieth birthday? No reason, actually, why everyone past forty shouldn't look and feel young and vigorous.

What I am going to discuss in these next three hundred

pages is the kind of information you'll find in few other books.

The facts about why premature old age is creeping up on you and every other person past his thirties (I consider any "old age" before the middle nineties to be premature) will astonish you by their simplicity and logic.

"In heaven's name," you break in at this point, "why hasn't somebody told me these things before now?"

I've no doubt some author has tried to impress you long before this with the need to "look to your youth." But the chances are the facts were not stated clearly or forcibly enough to convince you that *there is something definite you can do right away* to halt premature aging.

Every word in this book is designed to give you a simple, inexpensive common-sense program that should lift the burden of age from your tired, well-fed-yet-starved body like the touch of a magic wand.

Old Joe Jenks, and others like him whom you remember from your childhood days, were not freaks of nature simply because they lived long and vigorously. The truth of the matter is that Old Joe and other near-centenarians like him are actually throwbacks to those days when men and women lived prolonged, healthy, active lives as a matter of course— and not as the result of any whim of nature.

That "eccentric" nonagenarian you remember from your kid days was really a sort of relic from the long-ago era when the human race lived out its generously allotted span of years in vigor and usefulness.

What makes us so different today? Frankly, there are certain isolated groups of people on the face of this modern globe who do not age as quickly as the American Mr. and Mrs. U.

What I observed at firsthand during a tour of several South American countries did much to confirm certain nutritional studies I've had under way for a number of years on "how to cheat the calendar." We'll drop in on some of those amazingly youthful below-the-equator neighbors of ours a little later on.

There are no two ways about it—we just aren't living as long and as *vigorously* in this mid-twentieth century (despite insurance company tables on increased "life expectancy") as did the peoples of ancient times.

Perhaps I should amend that to read "you won't allow yourself to live as long and as vigorously." Not that you consciously set about shortening your life.

But you have been seduced down the dietary path to early and inevitable murder—murder of your youth, good looks, pep, radiant vitality and chances to live out a generous span of years. And the "murderer" is none other than yourself.

At first you may be inclined to raise a skeptical eyebrow at this accusation. But after I've finished supplying the facts to support my charge, whether or not you choose to accept the evidence and return an indictment against yourself as the unwitting murderer of your own youthfulness is your democratic privilege.

Yet the reader who accepts his own guilt and sentences himself to immediate corrective measures is the person who is going to feel and actually *look* a whole lot younger this time next year than his calendar age!

Chapter 2

HOW OLD IS "OLD?"

EXACTLY how old is "old"? At what precise spot on the calendar does youth end and old age begin?

We've all seen automobiles of "vintage" dates whose owners give them such careful, loving treatment (far more careful, in most instances, than they give their own bodies) that these conscientiously shined-up old buses perk along merrily for years.

While it's true that these venerable autos don't have quite the same dash and class as today's sleek models, yet, ironically enough, there are not infrequent occasions when these antique models are seen blithely chugging past their streamlined and *stalled* mechanical descendants.

Then we all know the fellow who buys a handsome new car—all bright paint and shiny chrome—and has it looking and running like a wreck in six months.

So there you have it—one car still in service and going strong despite the many, many years of license plates that have adorned its out-of-date chassis; and the other car, not a year out of the factory, ready for the junk yard.

The same thing holds true for the human machine. The sluggish, half-alive person who moves through each day with no more effort than absolutely necessary, for all his scant twenty, thirty or forty years on this planet, is literally *older* than the peppy man or woman past forty who wakes up each day with a genuine interest in what life is to hold for him or her in the next twenty-four hours.

Have you ever given any serious thought to the difference between living and being *alive?* That section of living tissue from a chicken heart kept for a number of years in a jar by the famous Dr. Alexis Carrel was not *alive*—it did not run about the barnyard, enjoying to the fullest its God-given faculties as a chicken. Likewise, the man in a coma lives, but he is not *alive.*

Staying young means living with vitality, in a body surging with power and energy, and with a mind tuned in to the vital principles of happiness.

If you're not alive to all the powers that are yours as a living, thinking human being, then something is wrong with the *chemistry* of your body. You probably know several persons of your same age who are far more alive and youthful than you are.

The psychologist would probably say that this difference in the ability of two persons to remain keenly alive to their surroundings and to their possibilities is a matter of "individual temperament." But I say that it's primarily a matter of body chemistry.

So-called "temperament" is chiefly a question of how well or how poorly your endocrine glands function. (More about them later as they enter into your eat-and-grow-younger program.) And the efficiency with which your endocrine glands function—or do not function—depends almost wholly on the *food chemicals* you provide for their intricately vital work.

That is why the sluggish person, of whatever age, who moves through each day with about as much energy and vitality as a snail in its shell, is probably killing his own pep every time he opens his mouth to drink or eat.

"Getting old" is not a matter of calendar years any more than growing older presupposes becoming senile.

Read that sentence again. It contains the concentrated wisdom of this entire book. It might well be made into a motto placard, to be hung where you could read it several times a day and ponder its truth.

Senility is pathological (diseased) aging. Senility is a breaking down of body, mind and spirit. Senility has no relation to the number of years that have elapsed since a person was born, because senility has actually been noted in persons still on the "safe" side of forty.

Premature old age is a disease—a *deficiency* disease, as real as pellagra, scurvy or any other human ailment arising from an imbalance in body chemistry.

What causes this imbalance in body chemistry? Improper diet, usually. When is a diet "improper"? When it fails to supply *constantly* and *adequately* the food materials needed to keep your body tissues in good health.

You may be sure a diet is "proper" if it is expressly planned to keep the tissues of your vital organs (heart, kidneys, lungs, brain, intestines, liver) healthy and in good repair, and to provide all the materials needed by your endoctrine glands for manufacturing their invaluable hormone secretions.

Then, with plenty of tissue-repairing and hormone-stimulating food in your meals each day, your body chemistry will be in balance, provided you don't also eat food that clogs up the system and denies adequate nutrition to your vital organs.

"But how will I know whether my diet is proper?" you ask with good cause.

That is where your Eat-and-Grow-Younger program enters. Every part of that program (see Part II) has been carefully planned to give you a proper, though still *appetizing,* diet which will nourish your endocrine glands and keep the tissues of your muscles and organs from becoming prematurely "worn out."

The chemical laboratory of your digestive tract converts the food you eat into still other, more readily usable food chemicals. You may not think of that sirloin steak, green salad and cup custard you had for dinner as being "chemicals."

But by the time those items reach your bloodstream, all resemblance to the food as you last saw it has disappeared. The steak, the greens and the custard have been converted, in the laboratory of your digestive tract, into the food chemicals needed by the living, breathing cells that make up your body.

We often speak of the human body as a "machine." Yet, actually, your body is more than a machine—it's an extremely complex laboratory where intricate chemical reactions take place which no human chemist has ever been able to duplicate.

The awe-inspiring thing about this mysterious body of yours is that when some "mechanical" part breaks down, more likely than not *under ideal conditions* your "chemical laboratory" can rush quickly produced substances to the spot that needs repairing, in order that life may go on and the body's efficiency not be seriously impaired.

You'll notice I said that "under ideal conditions" the chemical laboratory in your body can produce quickly those mending substances needed to put injured or worn-out body parts back in good working order.

What are those ideal conditions?

First, certain "test tubes" (the endocrine *glands*) must be in proper working order.

Second, enough of a certain food element known as *protein* must be provided the body's chemical laboratory, not only to keep the glandular "test tubes" themselves up to par, but also to rebuild constantly wearing out cells throughout your entire body.

These, then, are the ideal conditions under which your body, at any age, is given the power to renew your youth and prolong your vitality: *Endocrine glands in good working order, and an abundance of protein in the daily diet.*

Chapter 3

THE SECRET OF STAYING YOUNG

THE secret of feeling and looking younger than your years is really not a secret at all. It's not some witch's brew or alchemist's formula to be guarded jealously from the eyes of the unbeliever or the hands of the uninitiate.

Possibly the common-sense simplicity of staying younger than your years is what keeps it from being readily accepted by the great mass of our people, since we are forever inclined to depreciate simple truths.

We might go so far as to define the secret of prolonging youth and keeping youthfully fit as a kind of dietary golden rule: "Do unto your body as you would that it do unto you."

Prehistoric man instinctively followed this dietary golden rule. So did most of the ancient peoples, and some of our grandparents, while a few peoples on earth today still practice it.

During a tour of South American countries, I met some remarkable oldsters with a "talent" for living long and vigorously. In Uruguay and Argentina I noticed an amazing number of older persons whose pep and stamina was nothing short of miraculous, compared to that of the average American of the same age.

I was first impressed by these energetic older people in Montevideo, the completely modern, thriving capital of Uruguay. I was amazed by the unusual number of older persons stepping briskly about their business in the city streets as though life was important to them, and there were many things to be accomplished.

During my stay, I mentioned to my Uruguayan host what I had noticed about the uncommon number of vigorous, young-looking, older persons taking part in the city's daily activities. At first he was unimpressed by my observation, shrugging it off as of no scientific significance. But then he began thinking more deeply on the subject when I mentioned that in the more tropical parts of Brazil I had been singularly impressed by the lack of elderly persons to be seen on the streets.

"You're right," he conceded at length. "My country— Argentina, too—does seem to have more physically fit older persons than any other country in South America. Why, I wonder? Climate, perhaps?"

"More probably a matter of diet," was my answer, remembering the high-starch diets of tropical Brazil as compared to the meals I had noted being set before the Uruguayans in the city's splendid restaurants: plates containing liberal portions of meat, roasted or broiled; bowls generously heaped with green salads; and trays of temptingly arranged fresh fruits.

I had marveled at Uruguayan digestions that could eat with gusto foods and portions which ordinarily would have "appalled" the average American of similar age and circumstances.

It's a pleasure to remember the youthful glow of mind and body enjoyed by the grandmother of my host, a charming woman in her late seventies.

At the magnificent beach, Punta del Este, she swam in the surf along with her grandchildren and great-grandchildren! And after the traditionally late dinner of Latin countries, she joined in the dancing with the same eagerness as her great-granddaughters.

Nor, when the music had sounded a tango or a waltz, did her partners seek her out through any sense of duty, for this wonderful little lady, with her extraordinary pep and poise, danced as gracefully as any of the young girls on the floor.

I love to remember her, for she is what so many of our own wives, mothers and grandmothers could be at her age.

In Argentina, on an *estancia* not far from Buenos Aires, I had another close-up view of those oldsters whose appearances and abilities belied their calendar years.

My host was a wealthy Argentinian, educated in England, whose *estancia* was devoted to raising blooded horses for racing and for polo. His pastures extended for thousands of acres, and across them roamed large numbers of the finest horseflesh I've ever seen—and some of the youngest "old men."

Picturesque as was their garb, I was most attracted by their faces. For it was only by their faces that I could tell which were the older Gauchos, since all of them, young and old alike, performed the same arduous tasks. There were a dozen or more Gauchos on that *estancia* who were either nearing seventy or had already passed it.

"You're to be commended for keeping on those older fellows," I remarked to my host. "In my country they would long since have been replaced or pensioned off."

"Not at all," came his quick reply, "I'm very lucky to have them. They are the backbone of my *estancia*. Most of them were with my grandfather. My worry is what I shall do without them. But that probably won't be for another ten years or so."

"Surely you don't expect those old fellows to spend all day in the saddle when they're past eighty! Why, they must be slowing down even now."

"You think so?" He grinned at me and winked. *"Bueno,* tomorrow we'll ride with Justino, the oldest of the lot . . . he must be well past seventy. Then, after we return, tell me whether you still doubt that Justino and the others will be around ten years from now!"

The next morning my host and I were in the saddle before dawn, along with the past-seventy Justino and two of his colleagues. Our destination was an *estancia* some twenty-five miles away where we were to deliver a herd of horses.

Now, a Gaucho pony knows only two speeds—stop and full speed ahead. Rarely are they walked, and a canter and a trot are unknown gaits to them.

I am accustomed to an exhausting amount of physical activity every day, and it takes a lot to bring me to the point where I actually sense physical fatigue. But I freely confess that at the end of that day in the saddle—we rode close to fifty miles cross-country between dawn and dusk—I was more than glad to crawl into bed embarrassingly soon after dinner.

Yet down in the Gauchos' quarters I heard Justino and his confrères playing the guitar, singing and later enjoying a game of cards until long after I had gone to bed.

I no longer had any doubts that Justino and the other old Gauchos would still be around to do a hard day's riding ten years from then. Their vigor, agility and capacity for performing a full day's hard work was nothing short of phenomenal.

Nor were they the only such older horsemen I saw on the

pampas. Later, in my travels across the fertile Argentine plains, I encountered many more Gauchos whose actual calendar years would have made them long since eligible for "social security" in this country.

Before leaving the *estancia* near Buenos Aires, I took a meal with Justino and the other Gauchos down at their quarters. A whole sheep (sometimes it was a side of beef) was roasted in the skin over an open fire. When the meat was done to a turn, nicely browned on the outside but tender and juicy on the inside, large chunks were hacked off by each man with the long-bladed knife he wears at the back of his broad belt.

These large chunks of meat, followed by second and third helpings until nothing was left but the carcass, constituted the entire meal—no potatoes, no bread, no pie.

Nothing but meat, followed by a gourd of the brew made from the green herb called maté. Yet this was not an exceptional meal with them—it was the diet they followed three times daily, year in, year out. Meat is the sustenance of these people of the pampas countries—Uruguay and Argentina.

In the larger cities, of course, with the coming of American and European eating habits, more and more sweets and starches are being consumed. But the old-timers and the younger people living away from the foreign influences of the cities depend on meat alone for nourishment, plus repeated gourds of maté sipped at various times during their long day.

Meat, of course, is another way of saying *protein*. For meat provides the highest type, most complete protein.

Hence, with a super-abundance of high-type protein in his diet, the average Argentinian or Uruguayan instinctively provides an uninterrupted supply of *repair material* that keeps his body cells in good working order.

That is why he does not "age" rapidly as do his starch-eating brothers to the north. These men of the pampas retain their youthful vigor and stamina long past the age when our older persons are thought of as semi-invalids.

"All very interesting," you may comment, "but is it *good* nutrition, this meat-and-maté diet of your Gaucho?"

To which I hasten to reply with a big, loud *"Yes!"* Far better nutrition than is to be found on the expensively itemized menus of the finest epicurean restaurants in our cosmopolitan centers, with their dozens of tempting dishes from which to choose—most of them too starchy, too sweet or overcooked.

Good nutrition is not a matter of variety or a full pocketbook. Careful selection and intelligent preparation are the foundation of good nutrition. "Good" foods actually cost less than poor ones. Many an expensively provisioned table is tragically poor in nutritional values because of unwise selection and wasteful preparation.

The Argentine Gaucho with his meat-and-maté will never be a nutritional pauper. And this is a lot more than can be said for about 99 per cent of us Americans who have a seemingly limitless choice of starchy, artificial, devitalized foods with which to tempt our jaded palates and starve our prematurely aging bodies.

Remember, *it is the nutritional pauper who early loses his vitality and glow of youth.* Any person who surfeits his body with carbohydrates and starves it of proteins is a nutritional pauper.

Protein is the outstanding food element that determines whether you look and feel like thirty at fifty—or fifty at thirty. Whether your muscles coöperate, or cringe. Whether age is a matter of feeling, or years. *Protein is your best friend at mealtime.*

You'll meet protein in several different guises later on. But regardless of the form in which it appears on your plate, protein will be right in there pitching for you, striking out old age and pepping up slack muscles. Before you can hope to Eat-and-Grow-Younger, you must make a mealtime companion of protein, your "youth restorer" food.

When I first began lecturing, there appeared in one of my audiences a little old lady who was brought down the aisle in a wheelchair by her nurse. I learned that she had severely sclerosed (hardened) arteries, high blood pressure and a diagnosis of "coronary thrombosis." In brief, she had been told by her doctor that it was only a "matter of time." But her will to live was stronger than her weakened body.

"There must be a way to beat this thing," she told me, "and I'm going to find it! You've given me the first real hope. Tomorrow I throw out all that soft pap they've been poking down me for years. I'm going to have all the meat, and cheese, and eggs I want."

About six years later she stopped me one morning on the street.

"It worked!" was her greeting. "I've never felt so good in all my life. No more wheelchair for me! I get around where I want to go all by myself." She was having the time of her life and was an active member of an elderly persons' club devoted to having a good time.

Can anyone doubt that in her case the humble "secret" of how to eat-and-grow-younger worked real magic?

Chapter 4

WHO IS THIS FELLOW "PROTEIN"?

YOUR neighbors, your in-laws, your friends—none of them may care whether or not you stay young and vigorous.

But protein does!

Protein is a food element as vital to human life as oxygen. Yet how many persons have more than a nodding acquaintance with the word?

Many people are as mixed up about protein as was a member of an audience in a Midwestern city where I lectured not long ago.

I had worked hard to put over the urgently needed protein message to them, for if ever there was a group of persons who looked as though they needed to know more about the "elixir of youth," it was those tired, haggard, old-looking people who sat before me that night.

And yet I was positive that very few of them had reached any more than their middle fifties. They were still young in years, but even their spirits seemed to have wrinkles.

After I had concluded my lecture and stepped down from the platform, a man approached me—a man as worn and weary-looking as any of the others, despite his well-tailored suit and prosperous appearance.

"I thought you were against drugs," he blurted out, "but you're now talking for *protein!*"

Here was a man of apparently better than average intelligence, yet he could not visualize anything as vital to human life as protein, unless it were a drug.

Despite my repeated stressing throughout the lecture that *protein is a food element,* this man couldn't get his mind out of the drugstore. Yet, after my first astonishment at his distortion of my message, I began to look at the subject from his viewpoint.

Every few days when he picks up his newspaper or tunes in his radio or TV, he is likely to hear the latest word on "miracle drugs"—drugs that are going to permit mankind to live indefinitely, to bestow eternal youth on a pitifully eager human race.

My skeptical listener undoubtedly reasoned that in divulging the secret of how to stay young, I should have been talking about one of these "drugs." Naturally the build-up he had been getting via press, radio, and TV, didn't correspond to my message: that the "miracle substance of youth" could be found right in his own kitchen.

However, it's not the public's fault that "common sense is so uncommon" about a subject as close to the heart of everyone as that of staying young and fit. Even the medical scientists who should be leading the public down the road away from premature aging and debilitating illness are themselves often vague about the sensible way to keep premature old age from the door.

Why this inexcusable indifference on the part of so many physicians toward nutrition? Isn't it about time that a too-long-delayed merger should take place between medical practice and nutritional science?

Perhaps there isn't enough so-called "drama" about commonplace items such as meat, fish, poultry, eggs, cheese and seed cereals. As a public that has cut its eyeteeth on high-pressure advertising, we've been conditioned to value only the "unusual," the "sensational," the "supercolossal." Hence something like everyday protein foods, without a big glamour build-up, are all too likely to be "poor copy."

Protein is the safeguard of your youthfulness and good health. It is a preventer of disease, besides being one of the best medicines for numerous human ills. And here is what I consider the real nutrition miracle:

All the while that protein is safeguarding your youth and good health, preventing disease or curing you of an existing ailment, it is also nourishing your body with highly palatable, *good-tasting* food.

Nutrition teaches us that all foods are divided into four main classes: *proteins, carbohydrates* (sugars and starches), *fats* and *water.* Thus we establish that protein is a food, not a drug.

Protein is the basic raw material of all life, either plant or animal. The word protein is derived from the Greek verb meaning "I come first."

Protein is stored by nature only in *living tissue,* and in places where it is essential for development of new life—in the embryo of eggs, in milk needed to nourish the young and in the *seeds of plants.*

Here is a little chart to help you remember where to look for protein foods:

1. *Living tissue—meat, fowl, fish.*
2. *Eggs and milk—intended to nourish newborn life.*

3. *Seeds of plants in their natural state—cereal and seed grains, nuts, legumes.*

Protein is the chief building material of your body. Eighteen per cent of your total body weight is *pure protein.* For example, if you weigh 150 pounds, then approximately 27 pounds of you are pure protein that needs constant repairing, replacing and rebuilding—with more protein, of course.

If you were to analyze a single cell taken from any part of your body—a hair in your head, the tissue in your heart, the lining of your intestines, the muscles in your legs—you would find this tiny cell composed chiefly of *protein.*

And, like the parts of any constantly operated, non-resting machine, your body cells are continually wearing out, needing repairs or replacements. So what are you going to do?

Patch up your protein body cells with carbohydrates? Just try patching a rubber tire on your car with flour-and-water paste, and see how far you'll get!

Protein should be the featured food in your diet at all times.

When you don't supply enough high-protein foods in your daily diet to make certain that these vitally needed cell repairs and replacements can go on without interruption, you're inviting old age to take over.

In the laboratories, nutritional scientists and biochemists have proved that *a diet poor in proteins hastens aging in the human body.*

I could cite case after case of elderly persons, weakened by tea-and-toast diets to the point of imminent death, who have been restored to life and usefulness by gradually converting their meals to high-protein foods. Their weakened bodies gained new vigor, and their minds become keen and alert once more.

Nobody who has witnessed these recoveries, as I have, could ever deny that protein foods are truly nutritional wonders.

A grievous error has been committed for many years by some medical men who ban high-protein foods such as red meats and cheese as "too heavy" for older digestions.

Through this ignorance of the vital part protein plays in preserving youthfulness and maintaining life, such men have "prescribed" invalidism and premature death for many an older person who otherwise could have enjoyed many more years of an active, useful life.

Several things start happening to your body cells as the calendar years begin slipping past the forty mark. Biologists tell us that "aging is a matter of changes in your tissue cells."

First, the tissue cells in older bodies are less elastic, less resilient, less able to recover quickly from fatigue and injury than the cells in younger bodies.

Second, the active cells in the older body (especially those in your glands and muscles) gradually grow fewer.

Bearing in mind what I've already told you about the great *restorative* powers of protein on body cells (as evidenced by the case histories of those protein-starved elderly patients miraculously restored to life and usefulness), isn't it sheer logic that the more years you carry, the more repair material you need each day? And what is that "repair material" except *food protein?*

The more enlightened of our physicians today recognize how wrong it is to eliminate high-protein foods from the diet of the average patient. Yet there still remain the diehard doctors who cling to the out-of-date theory that certain ailments such as arthritis, high blood pressure, certain kidney diseases, hardening of the arteries and diabetes mean "cutting down on," if not eliminating entirely, meat in the patient's diet.

There is the case of a thirty-nine-year-old woman, well known to me, who developed rheumatoid arthritis several years ago. Weighing all of a scant 105 pounds, she had dieted strenuously for years to keep from getting fat; she had existed mostly on tea and dry toast. Since becoming arthritic, her physician had kept her on a no-meat diet, his reasoning being that meat was "bad" for her condition.

Although only thirty-nine years old, she looked a good twenty years older on the day she was taken to the hospital. A flagrant case of *induced* premature aging—induced by both her own senseless dieting and her doctor's ignorance.

Like most stories, this one has a sequel. Thanks to the common sense of the young doctor later in charge of her case, this woman began taking mineral capsules containing iron to build up her blood hemoglobin. Also, she was ordered to eat *three high-protein meals a day.*

When last I had word of her, she had recovered sufficient use of her swollen arthritic hands to do some sewing—and to wash the Venetian blinds in her home—all this in only three short months from the time she was carried to the hospital, a victim of extreme nutritional exhaustion.

But, as a rule, you *cannot* look to your doctor to help you stay young. He is a repair man, not a rejuvenator.

Your determined campaign to retain the wonderful feeling of youth which seems to be slipping away should begin with your *next meal*—a meal built around protein.

"How much protein? And what kind?" you ask.
Which leads us to the old riddle: How much is enough?

Chapter 5

HOW MUCH PROTEIN IS "ENOUGH"?

SEVERAL years ago I set out to answer to my own satisfaction the question of "how much protein is 'enough'?"

Using myself as a guinea pig, for eight months I gradually and deliberately cut the amount of protein in my daily meals down to a point which I knew to be inadequate.

Every twenty-four hours I would consume only one medium-sized portion of either cheese, eggs, meat, fish or poultry. And about once a week I would skip the protein meal entirely.

During the first several months after the experiment began, I felt reasonably well. That is, nothing to brag about, yet not exactly unwell in any recognizable way.

But I did notice that an evening on the lecture platform or a day at my desk writing would leave me feeling head-and-body weary.

This was the first definite symptom that all was not well with me, because my usual strenuous daily routines, either while traveling or at home, had never before induced in me this kind of fatigue.

All I wanted to do was to sink into a chair and remain there in an exhausted kind of half-stupor, too weary to read or to converse with my family.

About the end of the seventh month of my self-imposed protein deficiency, I began noticing that my ordinarily good appetite was no longer so good. Mealtime became merely a routine that I must adhere to because it was "time to eat."

My customary pleasure in people and events was also gone; I noticed that even commonplace little matters would irritate me out of all proportion to their importance. I found myself "too tired" to have fun with my two young sons. Any crisis, however petty, would find me without my former ability to make quick decisions.

In other words, I was not the man I used to be. If I had not been aware of the cause for my "slipping," I would have been panicked by that unpleasant discovery which many of you have already faced: *I was losing my grip on youth.*

The time had now arrived to discover whether or not, after deliberately sending my youth on its way, I could coax it to return by building up the amount of protein in my daily meals.

Within a month after starting to eat three high-protein meals a day, I could sense a marked change for the better in my disposition.

And not only was my zest for life definitely on the increase, but my face had lost its strained, weary expression, while the same daily routines no longer left me fatigued and chair-bound at night.

I hope that you, too, may experience that inexpressible joy of once more feeling like your old self. There didn't seem to be hours enough in the day for me to catch up on all the things I had been missing during those long months of wake-up-to-go-to-work-come-home-then-climb-into-bed-again.

This is what my experiment proved to me: "Some" protein is not *enough* when you have that not-exactly-sick, yet not-exactly-well feeling commonly associated with "beginning to get old."

Although I had eaten three high-protein meals each day for years, during the experiment my body could not fall back indefinitely on its protein reserves for the reason that the body cannot store protein as heavily as it can fats, sugars, some minerals and certain vitamins. When not enough protein is supplied in the diet, your body turns into a heartless cannibal and begins to feed upon itself.

When a protein deficiency exists, certain body cells are consumed in order to feed the more necessary ones. Not that the destroyed cells are unimportant. But cells even more vitally important to a living body must feed on those that can be spared, at least for the time being. *It is this continued form of protein cannibalism that is the real cause of disease, of premature aging.*

At least 70 to 100 grams (2½ to 3½ ounces) of protein every twenty-four hours has been established as a *minimum* daily requirement for the average person with a good digestion. But here's the catch in this minimum figure:

If your digestive mechanism is not working efficiently, you may receive the benefit of only 40 to 60 grams of the 70 to 100 grams of protein you are eating each day.

It's well to remember that along about the fortieth birthday, in many persons the digestive secretions tend to become less and less acid, meaning that the stomach acids become less able to digest protein foods thoroughly enough so that maximum assimilation can take place through the intestinal walls into the bloomstream. (Drinking *sweet* milk with meals, or taking baking soda and other "alkalizers" after meals, are sure ways of preventing the stomach juices from doing an efficiently *acid* digestive job on the protein foods you've eaten.)

More than enough is safest with protein.

The food portions mentioned below will provide a *daily minimum* of 75 grams of protein, that is, provided you can be certain that all this protein food is going to be digested thoroughly enough to assure complete assimilation into your bloodstream. These minimum portions of protein foods are listed merely that you may judge approximately how to double, even treble, this minimum protein intake to meet your own bodily needs.

By no means am I recommending the following portions as adequate protein for three meals. *These quantities are given for the sole purpose of allowing you to compare your own daily protein consumption with the absolute minimum for good health*, so you may decide for yourself how far above, or far below, this minimum standard your meals will average:

1 average serving of meat (fish, poultry included)
1 egg
3 slices of whole grain bread
1 pint of fresh skim milk (or its equivalent as powdered skim milk, buttermilk, sour milk, cottage or other cheeses)
1 serving of dried lentils, whole grain or seed cereal
1 serving of cooked green vegetables
1 green salad
1 serving of egg custard
1 serving of fresh or cooked fruit

There is no protein in air, in water, in a cigarette, in a cup of coffee or in an alcoholic or carbonated drink.

The one and only place where you can obtain this imperatively needed repair material for your body cells is from the food you eat each day. (Concentrated protein supplements are available to persons who, for some reason, cannot consume enough protein to supply their full needs.)

Even 100 to 150 grams of protein food a day (approximately double the arbitrarily established minimum) may not be *enough* to keep you from becoming a victim of premature aging. Why? Because we are not nourished by what we eat, but rather by what we *digest and assimilate*. The cells in your body are not fed by what goes down your esophagus into your stomach; cell nourishment must come from the amount of *wholly digested* food that is assimilated through the intestinal walls into your bloodstream.

The same portions of meat, eggs, cheese, milk and seed cereals that would be enough to meet your neighbor's protein requirements for the day might fall far short of meeting your own needs—and vice versa. The reason? Because, as mentioned above, your stomach acids might not be plentiful enough or strong enough to break down all the protein in these foods into the form of protein (amino acids) that can be assimilated into your bloodstream.

(Also, two identical steaks coming from two different kitchens will yield two varying quantities of digestible protein, all depending on the care—or carelessness—with which they are cooked. See Part II for the proper ways to cook all protein foods with an eye to obtaining maximum nutritive values from them.)

Although it's easily possible for every man, woman and child in this country to get enough protein for an optimum diet, recent surveys have disclosed the alarming fact that *the diets of from 60 to 80 per cent are dangerously lacking in protein.*

Because meat, eggs, cheese and milk are the most expensive food items, when the budget requires trimming these protein foods are either decreased or eliminated altogether in favor of low-cost starches. And thousands of persons, mostly women, eat little or no cheese, milk, whole grains or seed cereals because they're afraid of "getting fat."

It may come as a surprise to you to learn that *not all proteins are alike.* Frequently it's not so much a question of "plenty of protein" as it is a question of making certain to eat enough of the right kind of protein—of *complete proteins.* The youth-protecting value of the protein foods you eat depends not so much on the quantity as on the *quality* of the proteins you select.

In recent years you've probably heard or read about "the 23 amino acids." What this means is that all food protein is broken down in the chemical laboratory of your body into *amino acids.* Amino acids might be well described as the *traveling form of protein* in the human body.

From these amino acids, after they reach the bloodstream, your chemically efficient body proceeds to construct the kinds of *body proteins* needed to repair or replace the varying types of worn-out body cells.

To draw a comparison: The contractor who builds a house does not use sand, gravel and cement in the form in which these building materials are unloaded at the construction site. You wouldn't have much of a basement or a foundation if he tried to lay down the unmixed sand, gravel and cement in their original form. To obtain the durable material needed for your foundation and basement, the contractor must prepare concrete from these raw materials.

In like manner, the food protein contained in an egg, a piece of cheese, a slice of meat, a serving of milk, or a bowl of seed cereal is not usable by your body for cell-building material until it has been broken down into its separate amino acids, and then *reconstructed* into the hundreds of varieties of body protein needed by the many different types of cells.

Up to the present time, food chemists have identified 23 different amino acids in our food proteins—some appearing in one protein food, others in another type and so on. It is also known that only 10 of the 23 amino acids must be obtained from the protein foods we eat, since our bodies have the marvelously efficient power of being able to manufacture the other 13 amino acids, *provided* the essential 10 are supplied in each day's meals.

The truth about these various kinds of food proteins was first suspected when laboratory animals were noticed to be slowly starving to death on an exclusive diet of certain proteins, and yet thriving on an exclusive diet of still other proteins.

From these observations it was discovered that some foods are *complete proteins,* while others are incomplete. What this means is simply that some foods (the complete proteins) contain *all 10 of the essential amino acids,* and other foods do not.

You could live to a healthy, youthful old age by eating nothing except the foods that are complete proteins (witness the exclusively meat-eating Eskimos and Gauchos), whereas slow starvation, with the onset of debilitating diseases, would be the inevitable result if you attempted living exclusively on the incomplete, not wholly digestible proteins found in vegetables and fruits.

Nutrition experts usually classify protein foods as *complete, partially complete* and *incomplete.*

Lean meat (this includes gland meats, fish, and poultry), eggs, cheese, milk and sunflower seeds are complete *proteins,* that is, they contain all 10 of the essential amino acids in correct proportions for maximum human nourishment. Whole grain products, soybeans, legumes and some nuts are classed as *partially complete* proteins—meaning that their amino acids are *not* in balanced proportions to meet all body needs. However, these proteins are valuable "secondary" foods that should be generously included in every diet, particularly the whole grains; whether you use soybeans, legumes or nuts depends entirely upon your ability to digest them.

(The Eat-and-Grow-Younger menus provided in Part II are built around liberal use of complete proteins, supplemented by the partially complete and incomplete proteins. In this way, a high-protein diet is obtained without relying exclusively on meat which, although a valuable complete protein, is also quite an expensive item to be served three times a day in most American homes.)

Vegetables, fruits and some grains are classed as *incomplete proteins*. Corn, for instance, contains only 7 of the 10 essential amino acids, while cabbage has even fewer. Yet by no means does this lessen the value of vegetables, fruits and whole grains in your diet; what "incomplete" means is that you would eventually starve to death trying to subsist entirely on these low-grade protein foods. But these incomplete proteins can be used to great advantage in a diet as supplements to the high-protein foods.

(When I say that you would starve to death on a diet of fruits and vegetables, I can imagine you thinking, "But how about the vegetarians?" We'll get to them a little further along. Like many other things, there's more to vegetarianism than meets the eye.)

Each plant or animal food we eat contains a special variety of protein. For instance, vegetables contain types of protein that cannot be used by the human body, and which consequently are excreted by the kidneys. It may come as a surprise to many vegetarians to learn that less than half of the protein content of legumes can be utilized by the human body. Therefore, to obtain that *safe surplus* of protein so vital as a safeguard against deficiency diseases and premature aging, the vegetarian must consume at least three times more legumes in weight than would be necessary if he had no prejudices against animal proteins.

The closer a food protein resembles human protein, the more valuable it is for human nutrition. That is why we speak of high-grade proteins, meaning those foods that yield a maximum of protein nutrition in relation to the quantity consumed; and low-grade proteins, meaning those that furnish the body with only small amounts of usable protein.

To illustrate: 100 grams of meat protein (high-grade) are far more valuable to human nutrition than 100 grams of carrot protein (low grade).

A diet built around foods containing all 10 of the essential amino acids is a youth-protecting, health-promoting diet because it is a high-protein diet. If any doubt still lingers in your mind that a high-protein diet is imperative if you are to look younger and live out your allotted span of years (four score and more), let me remind you again that *you are made of protein.* Your blood plasma, red blood cells, hormones, muscles—in fact, every organ, fluid and tissue of your body (except urine and bile) are composed of amino acids.

As I often tell my lecture audiences: I wish the food chemists had been foresighted enough to christen these vital body chemicals with a name more descriptive, more appealing to the public than "amino acids." I would like to re-christen them "youth restorers," "body rebuilders" or "pep proteins." For that is exactly what they are.

Let me outline briefly what we know to be the direct effect of the 10 essential amino acids on the human body.

Arginine is called the "fatherhood amino acid" because it comprises 80 per cent of all male reproductive cells (spermatozoa). When seriously lacking in the body, the sex instinct undergoes a marked decrease in men and women alike, causing impotency in the male. (Such a deficiency is often associated with early loss of sexual powers in men not conscientious about proper diet.)

Tryptophane is known to help ward off signs of premature aging such as cataracts, baldness and sex gland deterioration; it is also vital to the female reproductive organs. Your diet must contain this form of protein if vitamin A is to be properly utilized by your body, since a lack of sufficient tryptophane will cause symptoms similar to vitamin A starvation (eye disorders, easy susceptibility to colds and respiratory disorders and general weakness of the mucous membranes).

Valine is directly related to the nervous system (one part of the body that really takes a beating as we grow older), and your diet must contain plenty of this protein if you want to avoid nervous disorders and digestive upsets. A person starved for valine becomes abnormally sensitive to touch and sound, and has trouble controlling his muscular movements.

Histidine is principally a tissue repairer, and is active in producing normal blood supplies.

Lysine, when inadequately provided by the diet, has been linked with pneumonia, acidosis, headaches, dizziness and incipient anemia. It also has a direct influence on the female reproductive cycle.

Methionine, if seriously lacking in the body, may cause hardening of the liver (cirrhosis), and nephritis (a serious kidney disease). It is also necessary to maintain normal body weight and aids in keeping a proper nitrogen balance in the body. (Nitrogen, a protein, is as vital to human life as it is to plant life.)

Phenylalanine is closely linked with the body's most efficient use of vitamin C. This means that not enough of this amino acid in the diet can result in susceptibility to infections, and to other diseases connected with insufficient vitamin C.

The three remaining amino acids of the 10 essential ones are *leucine, isoleucine* and *threonine*. Their specific functions in the body have not as yet been completely explored by the scientists, although it is known that these three amino acids play a vital role in helping maintain the body's nitrogen balance, that is, the intake of proteins and the discharge of wastes and dead cells.

All 10 of these essential amino acids, plus the literally thousands of different protein combinations manufactured in your body from the original 10 (the red coloring matter in your blood, or hemoglobin as it's called, for example, may contain as many as 576 different amino acid groups) must do an uninterrupted job of building, repairing and replacing, if you are to remain a living animal.

A red blood cell lives about thirty days. This means that every month a fresh, newly processed red blood cell must be recruited from your bone marrow into the bloodstream as a replacement for the defunct cell. The same is true of white blood cells.

Kidney, bladder and intestinal cells are constantly being lost and must be replaced if these organs are to do a good job of removing wastes from your body.

Skin, hair, fingernail and toenail cells are continually being destroyed and new ones must be provided.

Internal and external secretions (such as hormones, enzymes, digestive juices, tears, skin oils) must be produced without interruption in a healthy body, since these secretions are continuously being manufactured and produced each day in such extremely intricate body functions as digestion and sexual activity.

I don't know whether you've ever thought of it this way or not, but the fact remains that the sole reason why you eat is to provide your body with energy, and to assure your cells of enough protein for all the vitally needed repairs and replacements.

You may think you eat because you "get hungry," or because food tastes good, or because it's pleasant to share a meal with congenial companions. But actually you eat because your cells demand material (protein) for energy, and for repair work. A cell can't taste, and it isn't convivial! Therefore, Nature tricks you by your taste buds into eating, so that vital energizing and restorative processes can go on without interruption.

Please ponder this last fact for a few seconds—then remember it the next time you are undecided between a plate of high-starch foods such as white rice or macaroni, or a plate of body-rebuilding proteins like meat, eggs, cheese, milk or seed cereals.

Dr. James S. McLester, well-known professor of medicine at the University of Alabama and one of the pioneers in treating nutritional deficiencies, says: "If a man would enjoy sustained vigor and would experience his normal expectancy . . . he must eat a liberal quantity of good protein."

Good protein means, of course, a complete protein—one containing all 10 essential amino acids. Meat, fish, poultry, cheese, eggs, milk and seed cereals are "good proteins." Notice, please, that Dr. McLester specifies a "liberal quantity" of good proteins, not a bare minimum.

In order to make sure that you have the correct answer to the nutrition riddle: "How much protein is enough?" your safest bet is to eat more than enough. The menus compiled for you in Part II are designed to provide at least 100 to 150 grams of high-grade protein a day. This may be further increased by between-meal snacks such as those listed in Part II.

Getting "more than enough" protein is the only way I know of to make absolutely certain that you have bolted the door against premature aging of your precious body.

Chapter 6

"BUT I'M A VEGETARIAN!"

FRANKLY, I am not an advocate of vegetarianism.

However, I realize there exist strong religious convictions which reconcile thousands of persons to a meatless diet. And I have no intention of attempting to convert them to a meat diet (although I shall suggest foods that can increase the amount of high protein in such a diet without materially increasing the bulk).

All too frequently, enthusiastic vegetarians will convert

to their way of eating others whose health may actually be endangered by this low-protein diet, and who have no strong religious convictions to prevent their adopting a more youth-protecting diet. It is to these *fad* vegetarians that any efforts at conversion in this chapter are principally directed.

My wife told me not long ago of a couple who unloaded twenty-four packages of macaroni and spaghetti from their basket onto the checker's counter in a large supermarket.

"We're vegetarians," the woman said to the checker, evidently by way of explanation for this somewhat eccentric purchase.

That's exactly the danger point in most vegetarian diets. High-starch dishes take the place of high-protein foods. And the protein obtained from lentils, legumes, soybeans and nuts is neither a complete protein nor ample enough to counterbalance all the pure starches eaten to satisfy hunger. Actually, many vegetarian diets are nothing more nor less than biologically unsound, high-starch diets. How such regimens can promote health and protect against premature aging no one has ever been able to explain scientifically.

Generally speaking, vegetarians fall into three classes:

The first group includes those who live mostly on fruits and nuts, and regard all animal food as physically degenerating and morally debasing.

The second group objects to eating animal flesh, either for religious or moral reasons, but includes all vegetable foods, in addition to fruits and nuts.

The third group is composed of dieters known as "lacto-vegetarians," that is, they are permitted all vegetable foods plus milk, milk products and eggs, although no animal flesh, either because of sentimental reasons or because of a false notion that a meatless diet makes for better health.

In the first two groups—those eating nothing except fruits and nuts, and those eating these foods together with all vegetables—enormous quantities of plant foods must be consumed to provide even a minimum of the body's daily protein requirements. After a time, the human digestive tract is likely to have trouble taking care of so much bulk. (As a doctor from New Zealand commented to me while I was in Buenos Aires: "Man wasn't created with the digestive tract of a horse, so don't expect him to eat nothing but hay!") For this reason, many vegetarians find themselves suffering from various gastrointestinal ailments that would be relieved if they were to adopt a less bulky diet.

The "lacto-vegetarians" are merely non-meat eaters. Since they are obtaining a high-grade protein from eggs, cheese and other milk products, theirs is by far the safest vegetarian diet, provided they are careful to supply their bodies with the minerals and vitamins, in concentrated form, which they miss by not eating fish, poultry or red meats.

One prejudice against meat grew up in the old days when a mistaken theory was advanced that "dangerous and toxic effects of putrefying bacteria in the lower intestine" was a result of eating meat and meat products. Nothing, of course, could be farther from the truth. Any putrefaction that takes place in the intestinal tract usually results from half-digested starches in a digestive system that is overloaded with carbohydrates.

However, I still encounter vague allusions to a bodily condition called "intestinal intoxication" which is blamed directly on "eating meat." To those of you who are vegetarians merely to avoid this vague ailment, let me assure you that this condition has been much exaggerated, and has little, if any, scientific basis. So why bring on protein-starvation, with all its accompanying dangers to your health and to your desire to avoid growing old too soon, merely to avoid "intestinal intoxications"—a vague disorder, not scientifically established?

Properly cooked meats do not implant germs in the body, nor do they produce toxic conditions in the intestines. The hydrochloric acid in your stomach juices is so powerful a germ killer that by the time the digestive acids finish their job on the meat you eat, it is wholly bacteria-free.

Meat is the most easily digested protein food and is highly nourishing. To shun it for any reason whatsoever is to deprive the taste buds of unmatched pleasures as well as to cheat the body of a high-grade protein that carries with it valuable supplies of minerals and vitamins.

An interesting study was conducted some years ago by the Medical Research Council of Great Britain to determine the effects of flesh foods on the health and physique of two neighboring African tribes living in Kenya. One of the men conducting the investigation was Sir John Boyd Orr who later became director of the Food and Agriculture Organization of the United Nations.

One tribe lives exclusively on milk, meat and blood—a protein-and-fat diet. The other tribe lives entirely on cereals and vegetables.

It was discovered that the protein-eating tribesmen, when full-grown, averaged five inches taller and twenty-three pounds heavier, and had 50 per cent greater muscular strength than his vegetarian neighbor. The women of the two tribes evidenced similar differences.

It's next to impossible for an all-vegetable diet to provide your body with an abundance of the essential nutrients so vitally needed if you are to enjoy a long life, and a *youthful* one.

Time and again I have had the late George Bernard Shaw and Mahatma Gandhi pointed out to me as good examples of "vegetarians" who have lived long and vigorously. Yet here's the flaw in this argument: Neither one of these two famous characters were vegetarians in the strictest sense of the word—they simply did not eat meat. Both of them ate liberally of eggs, milk and cheese, thereby fortifying their bodies with high-grade protein.

If you do not touch flesh foods (the most concentrated source of high-grade protein), then by all means you should include ample quantities of eggs, cheese, skim milk powder, buttermilk or other sour milk products, and seed cereals in your daily meals.

Using skim milk powder liberally in cooked and uncooked foods is a splendid way of fortifying a diet with extra protein.

And when buying cheese, make sure it is marked "Natural Cheese," because certain so-called cheeses marked "process cheese" find their way into the kitchen under false pretenses.

Read the labels when buying cheese and other packaged foods. It takes some real detective work these days to penetrate beneath the disguises assumed by the numerous synthetic and devitalized items which masquerade under names commonly associated in our minds with natural foods. For your health's sake, be label-conscious.

If you are a vegetarian, and have passed your fortieth birthday, you would do well to consider this important physiological fact that has a direct bearing on your ability to live long and healthily:

One advantage of a high-protein diet is that you can eat less in bulk, yet be well nourished, whereas the average high-starch diet overloads the stomach, placing a severe strain on a no-longer-quite-so-young heart.

However, if you're still determined to follow a meatless diet, then at least let me urge you to adopt the protein-fortified recipes for meat substitutes that I've prepared in Part II.

I hope you'll weigh the evidence, pro and con, which I present in this chapter, and then ponder long and seriously over the irrefutable facts about the disadvantages of a *strictly* vegetarian diet.

I realize that most of what I have said may be entirely at variance with what you've been conditioned to believe about nutrition. Yet be fair to yourself. Take time to mull over and digest these facts before going on to the next chapter.

This entire program of Eat-and-Grow-Younger demands an open mind, an earnest desire to learn the simple truths about correct nutrition, and a willingness to work faithfully toward the goal of looking and feeling far younger than your calendar years.

Chapter 7

TOO MUCH STARCH IS DANGEROUS

FOR several chapters now I've been acquainting you with protein, and explaining *why protein is your first food need*.

From the need of more protein in the diet we turn to the necessity to cut down on starch. Too much starch in the diet can be extremely dangerous.

Our national habit of gorging ourselves on starch-and-sugar foods and guzzling soft drinks is doing more to make old men and women of us long before our time, and to weaken us as a nation, than any other single factor.

Please don't misunderstand me. I enjoy a piece of pie, a slice of cake, candy or a plate of spaghetti as thoroughly as anybody. But I recognize these artificial foods for what they really are—*dissipations, not nutrition*. I realize these heavy starches and sugars are life-shorteners, not youth-preservatives.

Life would be pretty dull if we always did what we should. Of course, you would be far better off if you never let another bite of rich, starchy, artificial food pass your lips. But you are going to fall from grace anyway—even as I sometimes do myself. And it's a whole lot better for your psychology— to say nothing of your opinion of your will power—if you are given a 1 per cent margin for "nutritional sinning"! That is why I always include a 1 per cent dissipation margin in my Eat-and-Grow-Younger program. But you must keep it the *margin*, and not your mainstay.

There is a proper time to sin on sugars and starches, but that time is not at your regular mealtime. If you feel that you have to munch on a piece of candy, or eat a slice of cake, by all means do so at very rare intervals, *between meals*, and far enough away from the next meal so that you don't take the edge off your appetite for the youth-protecting protein foods.

But never, if you wish to derive any benefit from this Eat-and-Grow-Younger regimen, include heavy starches *with* your high-protein meals. In the menus prepared for you in Part II, I have provided desserts that are both appetizing and nourishing. Their food values are calculated in that day's total protein nutrition, so if you sneak in a rich, starchy dessert (pure starch, no vitamins, no minerals and certainly no protein) instead of the ones shown, you'll only be cheating yourself.

Like many another blackguard, starch has several aliases. When he wants to work his way into the good graces of his unsuspecting victims, he assumes the highly formal name of *carbohydrates*. And when he wants to appear at his most tempting, he becomes *sugar*. But it is as *starch* that he is commonly known.

Artificial starches and sugars are saboteurs. They sabotage your youthfulness, your mental agility, your power to be a vigorous, radiant person, glowing with health and youthful energy. Stealthily they undermine your sexual powers. Like thieves in the night, they rob you of your good looks.

Unnecessary aging begins with starch addiction.

Yes, that is the correct word, for it is an addiction, nothing less. More than half the American populace stays on a perpetual drunk—a sugar jag. The ardent anti-saloon leaguer who points a pious finger at the village drunk, and then goes home to three meals a day of heavy starch dishes—pies, cakes, rich puddings, plus munchings of bonbons and gulpings of sweetened beverages—is as intemperate as the old soak who tanks up at the corner tavern.

Any physician can verify this overindulgence in starches as a true addiction from his years of experience with the cheating done by obese or diabetic patients who are supposed to abstain from rich, artificial foods. Because of their long-standing addiction, these "food tipplers" cannot refrain from sneaking a bite here, a portion there, even though their health —their very lives—depends on a drastically curtailed consumption of sweets and rich foods. Physicians have discovered that no chronic alcoholic going through "the cure" can invent more excuses for cheating than these starch drunkards.

I am justified in calling these cravings an addiction, because carbohydrates (sugars and starches) are converted in the human body into a type of sugar which, in great quantities, gives the identical "lift," or satisfaction, as that experienced by an alcoholic when he yields to his abnormal cravings.

The sweet habit takes hold with almost as tenacious a grip as do certain drugs. Anything to achieve that temporary feeling of energy and buoyancy, no matter how costly the habit may be to the body in the long run. The nervous system of a person continually starch drunk can be undermined just as surely as that of a chronic alcoholic.

But I must be careful not to give all carbohydrates a black eye, for like many villains there is also a good side to our bad man. The carbohydrates found in vegetables, fruits, milk, whole grains and seed cereals are *good carbohydrates* provided from *natural sources*. These foods also contain varying amounts of protein (something wholly lacking in artificial starches), in addition to valuable minerals and vitamins, and furnish a necessary contribution to your Eat-and-Grow-Younger diet.

It's only when carbohydrates wander too far from the "straight and narrow path" of good nutrition that they become harmful.

You're certainly not going to be advised to pass up all sweets in this Eat-and-Grown-Younger program. Instead, you're going to convert to sweets that, before long, will have you turning up your noses at a gooey cake made with white sugar and white flour. Not only are the flavors of the *natural delicacies* provided for you "fit for the gods," but they are sweets that actually help you stay young.

But first I want to make sure that you understand the character of the artificial carbohydrates which, I'll wager, have made up about 95 per cent of your sugar-and-starch intake for many years.

You aren't alone in this serious nutritional error, for it is an accepted American custom to serve a menu something like this: fried potatoes, meat, white bread, artificially-flavored gelatin salad, chocolate pie and coffee (sweetened, of course, with white sugar).

I am not quoting this as some far-fetched menu seldom encountered on a dinner table. This is a menu copied word-for-word from a recent newspaper article, describing the foods in the chow line of the enlisted men's mess at a large army camp in the East—a place where nutrition supposedly would be at its scientific best.

Yet there was white bread made of devitalized grain, a salad made with a gelatin that is artificially flavored and colored with coal-tar dyes and sweetened with white sugar (as are most artificially flavored, ready-prepared gelatin desserts), chocolate pie made of more devitalized white sugar and more white flour, with still more refined white sugar in the coffee.

No, indeed, we Americans need never worry about not

getting "enough" carbohydrates. Our danger comes from getting too much of the *wrong kind of carbohydrates.*

What are the "wrong kind" of carbohydrates?

Let's take bread as an example—the "staff of life." But is it?

Dr. Agnes Fay Morgan of the University of California stated that modern production methods rob bread of *30 nutrients.* Think of it! You are eating bread under the mistaken idea that it is giving you a certain amount of nourishment, yet it is 30 nutrients poorer than the bread your ancestors baked in their kitchens.

All the advertising hullabaloo about "enriched" floor, which began during World War II in an ill-planned, not-wholly-honest attempt to raise the country's nutritional standards, did succeed in restoring 4 out of the 30 missing nutrients, but still leaves you shortchanged of 26, provided your household depends on baker's bread, or you bake your own from *white* flour.

Which brings us to white flour, the principal ingredient of our nutritionally robbed "staff of life."

It might interest you to know that wheat has not always been the bread grain. Up until the beginning of the past century, in many provinces of France the peasants made their bread of chestnut flour. Other countries made their breads of rye, barley, millet and oak flour; while maize (corn) was the staple grain of the New World and still is in many Latin-American countries.

When white flour was first introduced in France several centuries ago, the powder merchants used only the finest quality of flour for powder to be dusted over the exaggerated coiffures of the dandies and aristocratic ladies. What a pity for the health of the civilized world that all milled white flour could not have been confined to this uncommon "outside" use, instead of being allowed to get inside to "gum up" the works.

Nature never created a white grain of wheat or rice, nor a white grain of cane sugar. Such improvements were left to the ingenuity of modern processors. To produce the "masterpiece" of white flour (enriched or otherwise), the mills sift and bolt out *three-fourths* of the minerals (plus undetermined amount of vitamins B-complex and E), leaving only the white starchy cells and refined gluten of the wheat.

So-called "enriched" white flour is but a makeshift—an appeasement of public indignation arising because of the commercialized ruination of good grain by stripping it of its natural food elements.

I frequently tell my lecture audiences to compare the

lunacy of preparing a fine roast, then throwing it away and serving the water used to rinse the roasting pan with the equal idiocy of milling the food values out of wheat, and then foisting the residue onto the public as white flour, a commodity that enters into every meal.

The same sort of criminal processing takes place with sugar cane and sugar beets which are milled and refined down to sickly white crystals devoid of all food values except pure starch.

White sugar is 100 per cent carbohydrate, containing no proteins, no vitamins and no minerals. It contributes absolutely nothing to your body except an energy which could be far better obtained from other food sources. When too much white sugar is used, your tendency is to neglect other more nourishing, youth-promoting foods.

What the processors do to rice and to corn is equally maddening. They strip off the outer husk of the rice, leaving a wholly starchy product.

If undeniable proof is wanted of the harm done to a people by a high-starch diet, I have only to cite our good friends, the Brazilians. For many generations, the lower-class Brazilian living in the areas near the equator has subsisted mainly on rice, bread and mandioca—all of them high starches—usually washed down by nauseatingly sweet beverages.

Life expectancy among these people has never been high, and they are frequently made fun of for a "laziness" that is actually a *deficiency disease* brought on by protein starvation. I have seen more than one of them lying sprawled out asleep in the street or on the dock, as though they had dropped right where they were at the moment when their extremely limited supply of energy gave out.

Especially noticeable was the difference between the vitality and ingenuity of the Brazilian stevedore and that of the dock hands in Uruguay and Argentina. The starch-stuffed Brazilian was lethargic, and slow to comprehend commands or the need for changing his routine; whereas the meat-eating Uruguayans and Argentineans who handled our ship and the near-by vessels did more than twice the amount of work, with a minimum of direction from their bosses.

Many of those poor, protein-starved Brazilian stevedores must have been men in their early twenties and thirties, surely none past their middle forties. And yet each moved with the careful slowness of a man who had reached the time of life when he must begin to show more consideration for aging muscles and brittle bones. There are none of the snap and zip about them that I saw in the dock workers in Montevideo or Buenos Aires. It made me tired just to watch the slow, I-don't-believe-I-can-make-it motions of the tropical Brazilians as they went unwillingly, or so it seemed, about their jobs.

Here in our own country, the National Safety Council warns automobile drivers against overeating on starches before and during trips. That stuffed feeling which is the sure result of a too-starchy meal (rarely can anyone eat enough protein to produce that gorged feeling, since the appetite is satisfied much quicker with protein foods than with high starches) cuts down your mental and physical alertness, and leaves you wanting to "doze," an extremely dangerous desire when one is behind the wheel of an automobile.

The average driver has the habit of stuffing himself on candies, cake, pie, sandwiches and sweet drinks, all easily accessible to the motorist at every roadside stand; often he substitutes these all-starch items for regular protein meals.

"One of the worst of the many bad food habits that Americans have acquired is their use of sweetened carbonated beverages." This quotation is from Drs. R. M. Wilder and T. E. Keys in the *Handbook of Nutrition* (American Medical Association). The soda pop addict is a ready victim of edgy nerves, irritability and hazy thinking, to say nothing of digestive upsets caused by the fermenting sugar in the liquid, together with its high artificial carbonization. The soft drink fiend can become just as jittery, just as much of an addict to his "lift" beverages as the chronic alcoholic or the drug user.

What is true of the eating habits of the average driver probably holds good for you and every other forty-plus reader of these words.

You bought this book because you realized you were losing your grip on youth—and that feeling of age probably got its head start on you because you always have eaten too much starch.

Let me turn clairvoyant for a moment, and "project" my thoughts with you through an average day's eating.

Your breakfast consisted of a fruit—perhaps a canned juice (sweetened with white sugar), or half a grapefruit liberally sprinkled with sugar. Your cereal bowl was filled with a dry, wholly artificial pile of something whose resemblance to a grain long since ceased to exist. And, of course, you reached again for the sugar bowl to flavor this already too-starchy cereal.

Toast?

Of course, and more than likely made with white bread;

or perhaps a sweet roll or two, well coated with sugar frosting, eaten with your generously sugared coffee.

"Please pass the jelly." More sweet. Some mornings you do get around to eating an egg, but usually you're too full after downing your starchy cereal and toast to want anything more. So off you go to work. You feel quite a bit less than up to par; but by now you're probably belching as all the breakfast starches, plus those left undigested from previous meals, begin fermenting in your digestive system.

By mid-morning you're feeling pretty pepless. So what do you do? If you're at work, you take time out for a candy bar, or a soft drink, or maybe more coffee and another sweet roll.

Then comes lunch. You're hungry—and yet you're not. How about a sandwich, a cup of coffee and a piece of pie?

That holds you until about three-thirty, when you begin to feel so worn out and dispirited that you realize you'd better get something to eat if you want to keep on going until dinnertime. More pie, maybe a piece of cake this time, a candy bar, or a soft drink.

By the time you drag yourself home and get through a dinner that is a repetition of all your day's dietary sins (white bread, sugared coffee, perhaps a dish with rice or spaghetti or macaroni, and a starchy, heavy dessert), you are more convinced than ever that you're getting old.

You can't think straight any more; your job seems to take more and more out of you every day; there's no energy left in you for leisure-hour activities; and you are sleeping poorly.

I could go on being "clairvoyant" and trace your footsteps to the kitchen before bedtime for that piece of pie which was left, or for a sandwich, but you're entitled to some privacy in your dietary indiscretions, so I'll leave you for the day, with your intestinal tract full of fermenting, half-digested starches.

If you are the average person, of sedentary habits or occupation, the chances are that you eat about *75 per cent more devitalized carbohydrate foods than are compatible with your good health,* and your desire to feel and look younger.

This estimate is based on the consumption in New York City. Approximately 55 per cent of all food shipped into that metropolis is either white flour or processed white flour products—all of them devitalized, de-mineralized and devitaminized. White sugar, and the products made from it, account for another 20 per cent of all food shipments into the city.

This means that the diet of the New Yorker (which is more or less typical of other cities and communities) consist of *75 per cent artificial starches,* leaving a paltry 25 per cent to be divided among protein foods and natural carbohydrates. Certainly not a safe balance for health.

If you haven't already figured it out for yourself, the chief reason why starchy foods are so popular with boardinghouse keepers and restaurant owners is that these foods fill you up quickly. And when you're well stuffed on the cheaper starch foods, your appetite is dulled for the more expensive protein foods in the meals such as meats, eggs, cheese and milk. There's more profit for them (but certainly not for you) in appeasing your appetite with the less expensive macaroni, rice, spaghetti, noodles, white bread and starch puddings than in serving you ample portions of tasty meats, fresh vegetables and fruits.

An old trick, yet one which many a housewife unknowingly pulls on her own family. Unknowingly, I say, because no conscientious wife and mother would deliberately pull this nutritional fraud on her family if she fully understood the harm she was doing to their health—and her own, too.

"But we must have carbohydrates for energy!" you say.

You are only *half* correct. While it's true that the sole function of carbohydrates is to provide heat and energy, what about the Eskimos who eat nothing except meat and fish—protein foods? Merely because they do not stuff themselves with artificial sugars and starches, must they be shivering, lethargic beings?

The Eskimo, far from being a slothful fellow who huddles into his skins with his teeth chattering like castanets, is robust, energetic and warm-blooded. In fact, it's only where our "white" civilization has brought in its white flour and white sugar that the Eskimo ever falls victim to our respiratory and intestinal diseases. Colds and constipation were the "benefits" of civilization which we bestowed upon the poor Eskimo.

How then, if the Eskimos in remote Arctic areas never eat anything except protein foods, can their bodies receive the fuel and energy which we are told carbohydrates provide?

Every human body has been given the power to convert amino acids into either body proteins or energy sugars. Actually, the type of *carbohydrate moiety* produced in the body from food protein yields more heat and energy than any of the carbohydrate foods you eat. Protein burns with a hotter flame, producing more heat and sustained energy than either carbohydrates or fats.

If it were true that carbohydrates conferred plenty of energy and body fuel upon those who eat them, then those Brazilian starch-eaters I mentioned earlier should be among the world's most energetic people—to say nothing about having a body heat that would not permit them to live so near the equator.

You get varying quantities of sugars in every food you eat. Even the all-meat diet of the Eskimo and the Gaucho—neither of whom ever tasted refined sugar—yields about 15 per cent natural sugars which break down to form glucose. Plants are nature's sugar manufacturers, and these energy sugars are passed on to the animals, fowl and sea life that feed upon them.

When you eat enough protein, you need never worry about getting enough carbohydrates. Your big worry should be not to eat too much carbohydrates.

Protein is a complete food; that is, you could live long and vigorously on an exclusive diet of protein foods. This is not true of carbohydrates. A great number of war prisoners who died in Oriental prison camps during World War II perished because they starved to death on an all-carbohydrate diet.

Not only do high-starch meals overload the stomach and place an unnecessary strain on the heart, they are also pre-disposing factors in many ailments and serious diseases that appear in the later years. Therefore, isn't it nutritional folly to clutter up the menu with so many carbohydrate foods?

Without alarming you unduly, allow me to cite a few pertinent facts and figures on the unholy relationship between devitalized grains and the increase in certain fatal diseases.

Dr. Haven Emerson of Columbia University points out that since grains were first milled (that is, since the protein, minerals and vitamins were taken out of the wheat) diabetes has increased 1150 per cent!

Corresponding increases have also been noted in heart disease, kidney disease and cancer.

High blood pressure has increased 250 per cent during the past ten years.

Anemia and appendicitis have also increased at an appalling rate.

These are diseases wholly unknown among primitive peoples who use only unmilled grains rich in all the vitamins of the B-complex group. Even among the Latter Day Saints (Mormons) of our own country, who are taught to adhere to sound, health-promoting diets, there are far fewer deaths from these serious deficiency diseases than among a similar group of persons elsewhere in the country as a whole.

There is good scientific cause for believing that too much

starch in the diet helps build up those unwanted deposits of cholesterol in the arteries (see Chapter 9), causing them to harden and become brittle to the point where a rupture brings on a fatal heart attack, or a brain hemorrhage.

Heavy starch-eaters are also more susceptible to sinus and respiratory infections than are those who limit their carbohydrate intake to the sugars and starches found in natural foods (fruits, vegetables and whole grains) and build their meals around high proteins.

Many persons who attend my lectures have told me that all symptoms of their asthma disappeared after they had eliminated white sugar from their diets, substituting honey and fruit juices as sweeteners.

One woman, whose life had been made miserable for years by one sinus attack after another, experienced complete relief from this painful infection after she eliminated all artificial carbohydrates from her diet. You couldn't bribe this woman to resume eating white bread, white rice, macaroni or white sugar. She also noticed that, since avoiding white bread, her long-standing affliction of heartburn after a meal had disappeared.

Constipation, a common symptom of digestive disorders, is another universal ailment that can be traced directly to high-starch food habits. The same holds true for gas in the intestines and belching, which are uncomfortable manifestations of undigested starches fermenting in the digestive tract.

Cancer, a dread word at any age and especially after forty, has been linked to *overconsumption of carbohydrates*. Chronic irritations and other causes of cancer, have less chance of stirring up riotous malignancies if the body is not oversupplied with carbohydrate foods.

This was postulated several years ago at the McArdle Memorial laboratory for Cancer Research, University of Wisconsin, and at Michael Reese Hospital in Chicago. A yellow chemical called benzpyrene, known to cause skin cancer was tested on 100 laboratory animals. Seventy-two of these developed cancer within six months—and these 72 were those that deliberately had been given 40 per cent more calories (in starch foods) than were needed for good nutrition.

The diets given the other animals, that proved highly resistant to cancer, contained a full quota of protein foods, yet totaled little more than half as many calories as were contained in the high-starch diets given the animals developing cancer. The same experiment was repeated many times— and always with the same results: The group of animals receiving *less carbohydrates* developed the fewest number of cancers.

This does not mean, however, that any person with cancer can cure himself by cutting down on the amount of high-starch items in his diet. Unfortunately it doesn't work that way. But the message to be derived from this research is that *limiting the amount of high-starch foods in the diet is possible insurance against developing cancer,* however remote it may be.

Here is the scientific reasoning behind the results of this cancer research: Biologists have good reason to believe that cancer begins with the formation of a single cell that is abnormal because it lacks *normal proteins,* or because of a disturbance in hormone balance, plus other reasons not yet fully explored.

During the so-called "critical" period of cancer development (this immediately precedes the stage at which the disease can be detected by either the patient or the doctor), the cancerous cells must compete with normal body cells for nourishments. If there is only enough food for the normal cells, then the cancer cells will be starved out.

This is true because, at the start of the critical period, the cancerous cells have not yet had time to establish their own direct blood supply, as they do during the final or progressive period. Since they cannot receive food directly from their own blood supply, cancerous cells must compete with healthy cells for the nourishment present in fluids brought to the tissues by the bloodstream. At this stage of cancer, the normal cells have a better chance of survival because they are still the more vigorous cells.

Growth requirements for abnormal, or cancerous, cells are quite different from those of healthy cells. For this reason, whatever nourishment is present will be taken up at once by the normal body cells, leaving the cancerous cells either to starve because there is no surplus nourishment for them— or to thrive because more food was taken in by the body than was needed.

If there is no surplus nourishment, cancerous cells must starve and die. But if there is a superabundance of body sugars in the tissue fluids, derived from too much starch in the diet, cancerous cells are assured all the nourishment they require to make them grow and thrive. And thus the abnormal growth may progress to its third, and final, stage.

Cancer is known to be more prevalent among people whose diets are high in carbohydrates. Among the Navajo and Hopi Indians of our Southwest, only 36 cases of cancer were found in 30,000 patients admitted to hospitals. Yet among the same number of white persons, approximately 1,800 cases of cancer would have been discovered. Why should these Indians have such strong resistance to cancer?

Diet seems to be the answer. These tribes do not overeat. In fact, their diet would seem extremely inadequate to us. Moreover, the Navajo and the Hopi Indians are *protein-eaters*, consuming very little carbohydrate. Draw your own conclusions.

I have singled out these ailments and diseases—heart trouble, hardening of the arteries, respiratory infections, constipation, indigestion and cancer—because they are commonly associated with the past-forty group. I don't need to emphasize that all these diseases and ailments are destroyers and killers in one way or another. Even those not commonly thought of as "fatal" can destroy your hold on youth, cutting down your physical vitality and mental alertness almost to the vanishing point.

It would be tragic enough if you had to depend on white breads, refined sugar, macaroni, rice and rich desserts to keep from starving.

In that case, no one could censure you for filling your stomach with these potentially dangerous foods.

But to deliberately destroy your youth and shorten your life because of an acquired starch-and-sugar habit, after being told all the facts about these saboteur foods, is one way of proving that you *want* to grow old prematurely and don't care what happens to your precious body.

Are the taste pleasures you derive from these high-starch foods worth the heavy cost to you in health and good looks?

Think it over.

Chapter 8

THESE EIGHT DETERMINE YOUR AGE

BEN BALD treats his thinning hair to a series of expensive scalp treatments, while Susie Sallow spends plenty of hard-earned money for creams and lotions advertised as "rejuvenating" sallow, wrinkled skins. Both of them are deluded into attempting these costly, last ditch measures for regaining a youthful appearance because they believe that the hair and the skin can be "nourished" from the outside. Nothing could be farther from the truth!

For by the time these signs of premature age show up on the outside, you may be sure that you've also started to age quite a bit on the inside. A youthful appearance begins inwardly—with healthy, properly nourished endocrine glands.

Before my efforts to help you recover your lost youth can progress any further, you must realize that these endocrine glands of yours are the *dictators* which determine whether or not your all-out campaign to look and feel younger will succeed or fail.

There's no denying that some of us are born with healthier glands than others. Yet the fact remains that even an ordinarily healthy set of glands can be neglected and ill-nourished to the point of beginning the aging process years before it normally should set in.

Your glands must be nourished with the proper food elements or you can't depend on them to lend you much aid in the effort to regain your vanishing youth.

If a part of the human body could be described as "temperamental," then I would say the word was coined to fit our endocrine glands and their hair-trigger sensitivity. They hold unlimited power over every human being, keeping one person young and vigorous despite the passing years, condemning another to a premature old age and thrusting a third into a morass of depressed thoughts and nagging ill health.

The names of these eight glandular despots are *pituitary, thyroid, adrenals, pancreas, thymus, pineal, parathyroids* and *gonads.*

Eight strange names that mean all the difference in the world between life and death, happiness and misery, youth and old age.

How do these eight glands hold such vast control over your life? *Hormones* are the answer—a word that has become headline news in recent years.

When it came time to name the secretions of these all-powerful endocrine glands, some imaginative scientist chose the appropriate Greek verb "hormon," meaning "excite." For that, in brief, is the intended function of all hormones— to *excite* your bodily organs into performing at maximum efficiency so you may possess all the vitality, all the magnetism, all the radiance of a healthy, happy person.

Each one of the endocrine group empties its precious hormones directly into the bloodstream without the ducts (tubes) which characterize most other body glands. For this reason you may often see the endocrines referred to as the "ductless" glands.

No person can say with authority that any one of these glands is the "most important," because every one of the group has its work so closely tied in with that of the other seven that a slight upset in one member of the endocrine family reacts almost immediately on the efficiency of the others. What one gland does, or does *not* do, is registered without fail in the activities of the entire clan.

Unlike your digestive tract which can rebel with pains and rumblings because of the ill treatment suffered at your hands (with a knife and fork in them), your endocrine glands *suffer in silence*.

The only way you can tell when your glands are not functioning up to par is when you begin noting the *effects* of their suffering. These effects often put in an appearance in spots quite remote from the seat of the original trouble.

For instance, the two adrenal glands (each about as large as a bean) are suspended one above each kidney. Yet when these adrenal glands are not behaving as they should, the skin becomes dark and sallow, with deep lines. Note, please, that the adrenals don't advertise their upset by a pain in the small of the back where they are located. Instead, the warning signs show up in a wrinkled, sallow, deeply discolored skin.

As a further example of the devious ways in which the endocrine glands proclaim their unhappiness, there is the unpredictable thyroid, located at the front of the neck. Frequently any change in the normal functioning of this well-known gland may bring on ulcers in the stomach, or in the upper intestine.

The pituitary gland, located behind the nose at the base of the brain, if seriously starved or injured, may cause you to lose all sexual power, since the sex glands (gonads) in men and women alike receive their impulses from the pituitary.

Here is the outstanding fact about this group of glands which you need to keep uppermost in your mind as you sit down to the table at your next meal: *Your endocrine glands, as well as their youth-giving hormones, are made of protein.*

Protein foods are hormone builders and conditioners. Therefore, a continued lack of high-grade food protein in your diet can weaken these glands so seriously that old age has gained a head start on you almost before you realize it. Feed your glands—not your stomach—if you want to look and feel younger than the calendar says you are.

Nor is protein the only item on the "menu" for your en-

docrine glands. Foods—or concentrated diet supplements—
that provide you with all the *minerals* and *vitamins* essential
to keep a body glowing with health are likewise "musts" in
your program for feeding your glands.

Let's take time for a simplified "close-up" on each gland as
it relates to your goal of Eat-and-Grow-Younger.

The Pituitary, Your "Boss" Gland

The pituitary is no larger than a small-sized pea and lies
at the base of the brain, immediately behind the root of your
nose. The pituitary is the gland that bosses all the other
glands, and helps keep them on the job.

Although one of the smallest of the group, the pituitary
is the hardest-working of them all. No fewer than *12 different
hormones* are secreted by this master gland, meaning that
the pituitary has at least a dozen different tasks to perform
for your body.

Despite its miniature size, the pituitary is divided into two
distinct parts, called *lobes* (anterior and posterior), each of
which is a separately functioning organ.

To simplify the many and complex functions of the two
pituitary lobes, it's sufficient for you to have this summary,
showing some of the blessings bestowed upon you by a
healthy, properly nourished pituitary gland:

1. Normal blood pressure
2. Good muscular tone
3. Sturdy bones
4. Normal nerve tension
5. Efficient senses of sight, sound and smell
6. Normal flow of urine
7. Plenty of initiative
8. Zest for work and play
9. Sustained interest in life
10. Vigorous sex tone
11. Prolonged youthfulness

Whenever you see a person in the eighties or nineties whose
youthful appearance belies his or her calendar years, and
whose enthusiasm for living remains keen, you may be sure
that this person has a healthy, well-nourished pituitary gland.

Dr. Herman H. Rubin, distinguished gland specialist, says
of the pituitary: "While the thyroid makes available the supply
of crude energy by speeding up cellular processes, *the pituitary*

is responsible for the transformation, expenditure and conversion of that energy into healthful, youthful vitality."

Many persons are the nervous, worrying type because their pituitary gland does not produce enough of the special hormones that feed the brain. Such persons are likely to become quite irascible, especially toward those closest to them.

The pituitary gland, through the little-known *hypothalamus* that lies directly above it, is also the appetite center and the sleep center of the body. Loss of appetite and insomnia! Two universal complaints found in thousands of the past-forty group who have strayed from the rules of good nutrition.

Exhaustive research has discovered that the pituitary is extremely sensitive to diet.

If you do not eat enough high-protein foods (meat, especially, seems to have a stimulating effect on this gland), then your pituitary cannot produce a normal supply of its own dozen or more vitally needed hormones which, themselves, are made of protein.

In addition to protein, the pituitary is stimulated by vitamin E (richest food source is wheat germ); and increased amounts of vitamin A either in foods or in concentrated form, have directly beneficial effects on the entire endocrine group.

Also essential to a healthy pituitary gland is the mineral *manganese*. Foods rich in this mineral are citrus fruits, outer coatings of grains, green leaves of edible plants, egg yolk and all fish, especially those from salt water.

It might be well to mention here that a derangement of the posterior (back) lobe of the pituitary gland can cause an abnormal craving for sweets.

And again we see the old vicious circle beginning to form —too many starches and sweets, and too little protein resulting in a starved, deranged pituitary gland; and then a still greater craving for more and more of the same high-starch foods that caused the trouble in the first place.

Your Thyroid Sets the Pace

This well-known member of the endocrine family is located in the front of the neck. (A goiter is nothing more than a greatly enlarged thyroid gland.) The thyroid is larger in women than in men, and becomes still larger during adolescence, menstruation, pregnancy and menopause.

Thyroxine, the hormone secreted by the thyroid gland, is about 60 per cent iodine. This vital hormone is formed when organic iodine combines in the thyroid gland with an amino acid (protein), assisted by still another amino acid.

From this, we establish the fact that *protein is essential to a healthily functioning thyroid gland.*

Chief task of the thyroid hormone is to determine the speed at which you live—in other words, the rate at which your body consumes its oxygen. For this reason, the thyroid gland has the power to increase your sensitivity to all normal mental and physical stimuli. To an astonishing degree, the thyroid also governs the constantly changing flow of your emotions.

When functioning normally, the thyroid helps to keep you from becoming either too fat, or too thin.

Texture and quality of your skin and hair is regulated by the thyroid hormone. Surest symptoms of too little thyroxine in the blood are dry, coarse, goose-pimply skin; and dry, lifeless, brittle hair.

The thyroid gland is also closely linked with the normal functioning of all other glands in your body. Because the thyroid gives your body much of its energy and virility, serious interference with the work of this gland causes the sex glands to slow down, even to lose all functioning powers. That is why the sex instinct is very often dormant in a grossly overweight man or woman—their abnormally fat bodies may bespeak a diseased thyroid gland.

From the foregoing, you can begin to appreciate that the thyroid gland determines to a marked degree how youthfully attractive you are—and remain.

Since the thyroid hormone helps regulate the texture of your skin and hair, controls your weight, determines the amount of energy you possess and stimulates your sexual powers, it's no exaggeration to say that *the first outward signs of premature old age have their beginning in an under-par thyroid gland.*

When secreted in normal amounts, the thyroid hormone helps you stay mentally alert and physically attractive—two attributes that comprise the very essence of youth.

A healthy, properly nourished thyroid gland is especially important to the woman who is either approaching, or going through, her menopause. The thyroid hormone helps combat the overweight, dullness and apathy that commonly afflict a woman during this emotionally trying period. A serious decrease in the thyroid hormone at this time is also known to bring on arthritis.

A normal thyroid gland can also help maintain sexual desire in a woman during the menopause, and for years after she has passed through her climacteric. The same holds true for sexual power in men, who must also undergo a climacteric that usually sets in from about fifty to fifty-five.

I don't need to dwell at length on the fact that a normal sex life does more to help a man, or a woman, maintain a feeling of youth than any other single factor. And not only do they *feel* young, they actually *look* younger. The sense of loving, and being loved, brings a sparkle to the eye and a spring to the step that no other tonic in the world can bestow, whatever your age.

Protein has a specific and dynamic effect on all the endocrine glands, but particularly on the thyroid. This is true because protein activates the thyroid, keeping it from becoming sluggish, from atrophying.

Gland specialists tell us that the thyroid glands of senile persons are almost invariable atrophied.

Further, these same specialists say that keeping the thyroid gland healthy will prevent the dry and flabby skin, thinning hair, poor circulation, sensitivity to cold, easy fatigue, faulty elimination, lowered body metabolism and total loss of sexual power which not only are characteristic of old age, but which are also the unmistakable symptoms of an underactive thyroid in a prematurely aging body.

The foods necessary for proper nourishment of your thyroid gland include *high-grade proteins; iodine* as found in sea foods, in vegetables grown near the ocean, and in mineral concentrates; and *thiamine* (vitamin B-1) which is especially abundantly in millet and sunflower seeds, in all gland meats such as liver, heart, brains, in lean beef and lamb, in egg yolk, sardines, fish roe, codfish and chicken, together with whole grains, fresh fruits and vegetables.

If there is any doubt at all in your mind about obtaining generous amounts of either *iodine* or *thiamine* in your diet (the soil in which foods are grown determines the actual quantities of a mineral or a vitamin available to you), then I would advise supplementing your meals with these two nutrients in concentrated form.

Your thyroid gland needs both these food elements too urgently for you to "guess I'm getting enough."

The Adrenals, Your Glands of Survival

These bean-sized glands are located one above each kidney; they are called your "emergency glands."

It is *adrenalin,* one of their hormones, that spurs every nerve and muscle into immediate, perfect coördination when you face a crisis or a great danger. That split-second leap to safety from the path of a speeding auto; that burst of energy to save a loved one in peril—these are the kinds of super-human reactions which adrenalin gives you.

When adrenalin is poured into the bloodstream from your adrenal glands at the moment that some emergency message is telegraphed to them by your brain, your entire nervous and muscular system grows tense, prepared for instantaneous action. Your brain becomes more alert; your senses of sight and hearing become acute; your heart beats more rapidly; your breathing becomes faster; and your blood pressure rises.

As an added safeguard during any emergency, adrenalin sends continuous supplies of quick-burning glucose as fuel for your greatly speeded-up heart muscle. Then, after the crisis is over, the thick outer part of the adrenals, called the *cortex,* immediately takes command and calms down all the organs which adrenalin had excited into great bursts of super-human activity.

Healthy adrenal glands are one of the most effective beauty aids you could desire, since the color and quality of the skin is one indication of the way in which your adrenal glands are performing. A clear, rosy color usually indicates properly functioning adrenals; whereas dark, sallow skin, heavily lined, should warn you that all is not well with them.

The adrenal glands also have a lot to do with helping your hair remain young. The cortex is suspected of being the culprit when your hair starts to become gray, since the pig-ment which colors hair is partially formed and stored in this outer layer of the adrenal glands. Obviously, sluggish adrenals would more than likely be unable to provide enough pigment to keep your hair colored, and this "rationing" of normal pigment would result in faded or gray hair.

This pair of little glands also helps neutralize any poisons that may sneak into your bloodstream—and believe me there are hundreds of them waiting to destroy you every second of your life.

A disease such as blood poisoning or influenza, as well as surgical operations, places such heavy demands on the adrenal glands to "clean up" the bloodstream that the glands after-wards become weary, and their hormone secretions fall far below normal. That is one reason why acute nervous symp-toms or severe physical exhaustion nearly always follow a surgical operation or a serious illness.

The hormone that controls your amount of pep, as well as your ability to fight off disease, is called *cortin;* it is secreted by the cortex (outer layer) of the adrenals. Even a mild upset of the adrenals will cause lack of pep, and what is mistaken for "plain laziness."

So beware! Whenever you tire too easily and seem to need more than seven or eight hours' sleep night after night, then the chances are you may be suffering from what is called *hypo-adrenia*.

Other common warning signs of this glandular disturbance are cold hands or feet, and low blood pressure. Along with this mistakenly called "physical laziness" comes a marked mental lethargy that leaves you unable to think clearly, or to concentrate on important matters.

Since poorly functioning adrenal glands are certain to make you lose your youthful appearance and to expose you to chronic disease, you'd be well advised to pamper these two bean-sized glands—that is, if you don't relish the idea of an early, ailing old age.

The adrenals, particularly the cortex, are also *the first glands to be damaged by malnutrition*.

A lot of intensive research has been done in recent years on the effect of diet on hormone production, especially the hormones secreted by the adrenals. The conclusions reached were that through *proper diet it is quite possible to renew the vitality of the adrenal glands*.

Protein, together with vitamin C, seems to have the most beneficial effect on the adrenal glands. This is true because high-protein diets have been found to be the best measure for successfully combating hypo-adrenia—the ailment that keeps your blood pressure too low, your hands and feet like ice, and your mind and muscles about as peppy as those of a sloth.

The adrenals themselves have a very high content of vitamin C. Since we know that vitamin C is used in large doses to help combat infections, the conclusion now is that this vitamin helps stimulate the adrenal glands into producing more *cortin*, the hormone that fights off disease.

Because this pair of glands was designed by nature to pour forth adrenalin in times of physical danger, or emotional crisis, continued mental or emotional tension overworks your "emergency glands" to the point where your nerves and vital organs are constantly kept keyed-up to fever pitch owing to too many fake "emergency" messages from the brain, thereby sending the powerful adrenalin hormone shooting into your bloodstream when it isn't actually needed.

In times of stress, the adrenal glands also release into your bloodstream a substance called cholesterol (the waxy substance now blamed as a contributing factor leading to hardening of the arteries. See Chapter 9).

For this reason, many doctors believe that arteriosclerosis, and other "diseases of age" such as coronary thrombosis and cerebral hemorrhage, may develop as a result of this constant overstimulation of the adrenal glands by high-tension living, and day-in-day-out mental or emotional strain.

This emergency function of the adrenals to act as a powerful stimulant upon the organs of the body is a holdover from the days when man needed instantaneous physical and mental reserves to save himself from animal or human enemies.

But today, when most of our emergencies are chiefly emotional or mental, this continued outpouring of the high-powered adrenalin into your bloodstream causes the heart and blood vessels to take a fearful beating.

And because adrenalin is continually being squirted into the blood under the stress and strain of our highly emotional civilization, cortin is likewise constantly needed in big doses to get the body machine slowed down to normal again.

Since we know that the adrenal glands use vitamin C to manufacture the cortical hormone, it's not difficult to understand that continued high-tension living (either physical, mental or emotional) uses up a lot of vitamin C and releases a lot of cholesterol into the bloodstream.

The result is depleted vitamin C reserves—(unless special attention is given to replacing this vitamin through the diet)—with an increased tendency to infection (witness how easily an epidemic of influenza knocks over its victims during times of a local or national crisis).

It can contribute to and aggravate high blood pressure and hardening of the arteries. That surplus amount of cholesterol from the overstimulated adrenals has to land some place, and where more convenient than on the walls of your arteries where it clogs the free flowing of the blood, causing the arteries to "harden"?

If you want to feel and look younger than you are, you'd better stop setting off those mental and emotional "false alarms" that keep your body wound up as tight as a main spring.

The old proverb that "worry kills more people than cannons" was unconsciously aimed right at the adrenal glands, since the unwise use of their powerful hormone by an emotionally unstable mind is equivalent to killing off your youth —yourself as well—by inches.

A final word of advice on the care of your adrenal glands: Feed them plenty of *high-grade protein;* provide them with ample vitamin C (best sources are citrus fruits, melons, rose hips, apricots, strawberries, green vegetables, and particularly tomatoes). Make sure that foods rich in *Vitamins A* and *B-complex* are eaten at least twice a day. Provide them with the minerals *magnesium* and *silicon* (richest sources are citrus and other fruits, green and leafy vegetables, yellow vegetables, walnuts and egg yolk).

The Pancreas, Your Insulin Factory

To impress you with the importance of this endocrine gland, I need only mention the word "diabetes." Although diabetes was for years blamed on the kidneys, medical science has discovered that this stealthy disease actually starts in the pancreas, that is, *after* the pancreas falls down on the job of secreting *insulin*, one of its hormones.

When not enough insulin is produced, the bloodstream becomes overcharged with sugar. Insulin helps the body "burn" its sugar, converting it into energy. When not enough insulin is produced because of a sluggish or diseased pancreas, unused sugar lies in the bloodstream like unburned coal in a stove.

The quickest way to put your pancreas out of order is to stuff yourself continually with sweet and starchy foods. After you have committed this dietary crime for years on end, the pancreas becomes discouraged and gives up trying to produce enough insulin to burn all the sugar piling up in the bloodstream. Then, my friend, you have diabetes—a controllable disease, but definitely not curable, and a potential killer at any unguarded moment.

As though the job of burning sugar isn't work enough, the pancreas must also pour enough enzymes (substances that speed up digestion in the body) into the upper intestine to help digest starches and sugars before they can be converted into blood sugar.

From this you can readily appreciate what an endless task it finally becomes for the pancreas of the heavy sugar-and-starch eater.

If you want to show a little consideration for your hard-working pancreas, give it plenty of protein foods, since protein is necessary in the body to assure a normal production of the hormone insulin. The minerals *sulphur, zinc* and *chlorine* (found in green vegetables, all berries, fresh coconut, egg yolk, cheese—particularly Roquefort, dairy products, lean meats, salt-water fish, lobster, crab, mussels and shrimp) are all stimulating to the pancreas.

Three Other Members of Your Gland Family

The four tiny parathyroid glands (two on either side of the thyroid gland) are mainly concerned with regulating the supply of calcium in your body. For this reason, the parathyroids are an important quartet, since calcium is so vital to a healthy heart, nerves, muscles, teeth and bones—all of them your foundation for a youthful mind and body.

It's worth remembering that while controlling the body's supplies of calcium, *the parathyroids themselves need calcium to keep healthy.*

Hence, a diet poor in calcium is a two-edged sword: Not enough calcium for the parathyroids, which then retaliate by failing to produce the hormone that releases bone calcium into the bloodstream for your nerves, muscles, heart, teeth and bones. In addition to meat and eggs, the best sources of food calcium are found in dairy products such as powdered skim milk, buttermilk, yogurt and cheese.

The *thymus* gland lies in your chest not far below the thyroid. When you are born, the thymus weighs about half an ounce, then increases to almost triple its weight up to the time of adolescence, after which it begins to shrink again, until by the time you're fifty, the thymus is back to its original size.

The complete functioning of this endocrine gland is not as yet fully understood by medical science, although it is suspected of helping control the body's use of phosphorus and calcium, and of taking some part in producing white blood corpuscles, one of your guardians against infection.

Most mysterious of all your endocrine glands is the *pineal*, a cone-shaped little organ, no larger than a grain of wheat, suspended by a stalk just behind the mid-brain. Sometimes the pineal will shrink and fill up with deposits of salts known as "brain sand." This abnormal condition is caused by faulty nutrition, and recent scientific experiments have demonstrated that a *degenerating pineal gland will respond to a protein diet within a remarkably short time.*

The minerals potassium and sodium are also known to feed the pineal gland. Richest sources of these minerals are potato peelings (potassium especially), eggplant, celery, corn, green vegetables, berries, melons, black olives, citrus and other fresh fruits, lean beef and lamb, cottage and other cheeses, buttermilk and powdered skim milk, lobsters and oysters.

Your Sex Glands (Gonads)

I've left until last the glands which perhaps should rank first in your effort to retain the appearances and sensations of youth.

What qualities or attributes make people say of a certain man or woman: "He (or she) is so young for his (her) age"?

My first answer would be *sexual vibrancy*—for in these two words are contained the confidence, inward feeling of power, energy, vitality, enthusiasm, mental alertness, sense of attractiveness, assurance, stamina and radiant glow which are gifts to the young in years, and which may also be found in persons of *any age* whose sex glands are healthy.

If there is such a thing as "youth everlasting," then surely it must center in your sex glands, for they determine your youthfulness. The hormones secreted by the gonads (*ovaries* in women; *testes* in men) exert a tremendous influence on your physical health, as well as on your ability to retain a youthful appearance and to live a long, useful life.

Testosterone, the hormone secreted by the male sex glands, is the dominant factor in producing and maintaining a man's vitality, strength and sexual powers.

In brief, his *maleness*.

Female sex hormones, secreted by the ovaries, are *progesterone* and *estrin*. It is estrin that increases a woman's vitality and sexual desire; it is estrin that produces the femininity which attracts the male.

Although the chief function of progesterone is to help provide the best conditions for pregnancy, this second ovarian hormone also combats fatigue, irritability, insomnia, headache and backache—all of which are common female ailments, often brought on by an upset in the female sex glands.

A normal, happy life is next to impossible, unless your sex glands do their work properly. They are the real arbiters of physical and mental well-being. How young you remain, in mind and body, despite the remorseless calendar, is controlled mainly by your sex glands.

Sex and Diet

Several years ago a group of sexually normal men were placed, as an experiment, on a diet containing extremely low amounts of protein. Their appetites were satisfied with meals of high-starch foods.

Within a short time they lost all interest in women: bathing beaches, windy corners and ringside tables at night clubs held no special appeal for these protein-starved, yet otherwise normal, males.

Even mice, those useful little laboratory animals that obligingly develop human diseases and respond to human nutrition, will lose their fertility, go through an abnormally early change of life and become aged and decrepit if kept on diets low in protein. Yet when fed liberal amounts of the protein in *animal foods,* they enjoy a remarkably extended period of sexual activity, and develop no signs of premature aging.

Because we know that an extremely close bond exists between the thyroid and the sex glands, it's logical to assume that any continued diet low in protein affects the sex glands through a slowing down of the thyroid. One of the first symptoms of an underactive thyroid is decreased sexual powers. But when the thyroid is stimulated into again secreting normal amounts of its hormone, an early revival of sexual activity usually takes place.

In addition to protein foods, the minerals *iron* and *copper* are particularly important to the health of your sex glands. Rich sources of iron are beef liver and other organ meats like heart and kidney, dark poultry meat, lean beef and lamb, egg yolk, apricots, prunes, raisins, cane or sorghum molasses, whole grains, lettuce, beet tops, leeks and radishes. Copper is usually present in the foods containing iron, but especially in almonds, dried beans, whole wheat, prunes, calf and beef liver, shrimp and egg yolks.

And then there are the vitamins. *Vitamins and hormones are interdependent.*

Vitamin A, because it keeps all the mucous membranes of the body in good condition, helps your sex organs stay healthy. This vitamin also reinforces the functioning of the sex glands, especially the testes.

Thiamine (vitamin B-1), when insufficiently supplied by the diet, causes the pituitary gland to produce fewer hormones which stimulate the sex glands; this can result in seriously decreased sexual desire in men and women alike.

Vitamin D seems to have a chemical kinship to the sex hormones, and is known to increase sexual desire. The old "prescription" of oysters and eggs to strengthen sexual desire unknowingly took advantage of the fact that both these foods contain vitamin D, as do all fatty fish, tuna, salmon, sardines, cod and halibut liver oil. Sunflower seeds are an unusually rich source of vitamin D.

Many persons notice, too, that an outdoor life in the sunshine increases sexual appetites, and no wonder since the action of sunshine on the human skin oils produces vitamin D without the need to obtain it from food sources. Exposing portions of your body to the sunshine for a few minutes each day, so that the ergosterol in your skin may be converted into vitamin D, is one of the best ways to assure enough vitamin D for your sex glands. (Don't bathe immediately before sunning yourself, or you will wash off the skin oils, thereby losing this benefit.)

However, please don't overload your body with vitamin D capsules in order to stimulate your sex glands. This is one vitamin you can get too much of. Eat normally of the vitamin D foods, and try to get a normal amount of sunshine on your bare skin. During the winter months it may be necessary to take a small amount of vitamin D in a scientifically balanced concentrate.

Vitamin E is best known as an aid to keeping the sex organs in good condition. A serious lack of this vitamin may cause sterility. About the best food sources of vitamin E are wheat germ or wheat germ oil.

Hundreds of cases of so-called "impotency" in men, and "frigidity" in women have responded to diets purposely planned to provide generous amounts of foods rich in high-proteins, iron and copper, and vitamins A, D, E and thiamine.

Fortifying these planned diets with supplemental amounts of vitamins in concentrated form, along with the minerals iron and copper, often brought quicker and more lasting results.

You can't be any younger than your glands. And your glands can't stay young and healthy if they are starved. Foods that befriend your glands are the best youth-insurance you can buy.

Chapter 9

SIX COMMANDMENTS FOR A LONG "YOUNG" LIFE

YOUR great desire is to live a long, useful life, all the while looking and feeling far younger than your years. Certainly this is a goal worth aiming at.

But are you prepared to abide by the Commandments? Because everything worth attaining has a price. And the *price* of a long, youthful life is *planned diet*.

No more haphazard eating; no more pandering to a finicky appetite; no more plundering your body's health with indifferent and unwise selections of "substandard" foods.

At first, the careful and judicious selection of youth-protecting foods will be a novelty you'll enjoy. But after that may come the danger period when the novelty provided by a new regimen begins to wear off, and you are tempted to lapse into the "oh, it's too much trouble" kind of defeatist thinking.

Yet I promise you that once you have successfully weathered this period of temptation to return to the old haphazard way of eating, you'll subconsciously begin accepting, or rejecting, each food on the basis of its contribution to your youthfulness and long life, with the same skill as that exercised by a trained nutritionist. Instinctively, you will avoid the old "gooey" meals with which you formerly insulted your body.

The food commandments I am going to lay down for you are those that will afford you taste pleasures and adventures in good eating the like of which you have seldom enjoyed before.

While this book was still in the planning stage, I came across a published interview with Dr. Charles E. Dutchess, medical director of an Eastern research laboratory, and a scientist long interested in proper nutrition as the only way to attain a healthy, long life. His "six general rules" parallel so closely the health teachings to which I have devoted my life that I was elated to find a medical scientist speaking out firmly on the subject of "eating to stay young."

If you are already forty or over, Dr. Dutchess was quoted as saying, it is even more important to protect your body mechanism against the wear and tear of age.

And at fifty and sixty, and beyond, the six rules become still more vital.

The rules, in brief, with which Dr. Dutchess (as well as all nutritional scientists) earnestly seeks to acquaint the public call for "plenty of lean meat, eggs, low-fat milk, vitamins and essential minerals, obtained from a broad selection of meats, fruits and vegetables."

Let's take these six general rules—commandments I have called them—one by one, in detail, as they pertain to your goal of attaining a long, youthful, enjoyable life.

FIRST COMMANDMENT—HIGH-GRADE PROTEINS IN ABUNDANCE

The protein story has been developed rather fully for you

in the preceding chapters, so there is no need to repeat at length the fact that protein is essential for feeding, repairing and rebuilding your muscles, nerves, tissues, glands and vital organs.

In case of illness or convalescence, protein is the re-builder of your health.

Life insurance companies have an unsentimental, dollars-and-cents interest in keeping you well and alive for a long time. For that reason they issue a series of pamphlets and booklets loaded with sane advice on how to avoid illness and early death. I quote from one of these pamphlets directed at the forty-and-over group:

"An ample, nutritious diet is as important to adults as to growing children. Learn to like and to choose foods that are good for you. Well-balanced meals of vegetables, meats and fresh fruits are health-building meals. The impression that people in the older ages should avoid eating meat is entirely erroneous. In fact, some diseases are due to lack of protein which is contained in such foods as meat, eggs, low-fat milk and cheese."

The pamphlet then goes on to say that "older people die (aside from accidents and senility) only from *blood disorders, cancer, circulatory disorders* (heart disease, kidney disease or stroke) or *infections.*"

Let's see what nutritional science has been doing to fight these "disease enemies of your youth."

First, we'll take *blood disorders*. One of the most common of these in persons past forty is *anemia*. (See Chapter 18.)

The paleness which has come to be associated with growing older is often nothing except a visible symptom of nutritional anemia. There's no reason why a person shouldn't possess a healthy, glowing complexion in later years, provided his blood is rich with red coloring matter. But healthy blood cannot be formed without *protein* any more than it can be maintained without the minerals *iron* and *copper*.

Hemoglobin, the red coloring matter in the blood, contains no less than 14 different amino acids (proteins combined in as many as 576 different groupings). You can't build good red blood on tea and toast.

Because nutritional anemia is so widespread among all sugar-and-starch eaters, but more particularly in those persons past forty, I want to dwell a moment on this blood disorder which, in itself, does not kill, but which paves the way for more serious diseases.

[And I might add, as an aside right here, that although anemia may not kill you, it certainly does murder your youthfulness, for without pep and enthusiasm you can neither look nor feel young. And who can remain youthful while staggering under the growing burden of *anemia fatigue?*]

Anemia at any age, and particularly after forty, cannot be shrugged off as "not serious," for anemia in middle life is an ailment that can shorten your years of useful, vigorous living.

And certainly the mind of a person suffering from nutritional anemia is not equipped to cope with the bewildering personal adjustments that often must be faced, and accepted, after the fourth decade. If you suspect that you may be anemic, go at once to a reliable laboratory and have a blood count taken.

Let me point out that *unless anemia is checked as rapidly as possible, your heart ultimately will be damaged.*

If a blood count reveals that your blood contains too few red cells and has a low percentage of hemoglobin (that is, it is not red enough), then you should act at once to restore your blood to normal. How? By immediately converting to high-protein meals (those containing lean meat, liver, kidney, heart, dark meat of poultry, oysters, eggs, cheese, low-fat milk and seed cereals like millet, sunflower and sesame seeds); by eating generously of iron-rich apricots, molasses, prunes, raisins, whole grains, beets, parsley, radishes, citrus fruits and pineapple, to mention but a few of the foods with the highest iron content.

As a safety measure, your doctor will probably also prescribe a mineral supplement containing organic iron to rebuild your blood to normal as quickly as possible.

As an added iron tonic which you can prepare for yourself at home, buy some unsulphured apricots (usually found only in health food stores). If apricots can't be had, then the next best fruits in order are dried peaches or raisins. Put a handful of the fruit in a glass, cover with lukewarm water, stir, then let stand overnight. Next morning stir the mixture again, drain off the water into another glass, adding to it one tablespoonful of unsulphured molasses. Prepare and drink this iron tonic several times a week (the fruit should also be eaten). Also eat at least a handful of iron-rich, hulled sunflower seeds each day.

Because women, especially those nearing or passing through their menopause, tend to be far more anemic than men, this homemade tonic might well be used as a morning "pick-me-up" three or four times a week, while the sunflower seeds could form their between-meal snack.

Up to this point I have been speaking exclusively of simple, iron-deficiency anemia which comprises about 95 per cent of all anemia cases. But there is another type of blood disorder called *pernicious anemia* that was inevitably fatal until some twenty years ago. Even now, unless diagnosed during its early stages and treated immediately, pernicious anemia can be a killer disease. The most important thing I can impress upon you about pernicious anemia is the urgent need for an *early diagnosis*. Don't neglect the symptoms which, in their early stages, may resemble those of simple iron-deficiency anemia. If taken in time, pernicious anemia is controllable.

Another blood disorder is the inability of the blood to clot, meaning that a slip of the razor, or a kitchen knife, may cause death from loss of blood. Blood-clotting agents called *prothrombin* and *fibrinogen* are manufactured by the body from the food we eat, the principal nutrients used being *protein* and *vitamin K*. (This vitamin is supplied by green leafy vegetables, tomatoes, liver, eggs and rice bran.) The greatly lowered death rate from bleeding wounds among American fighters in World War II has been attributed to the high-protein meals fed all branches of the service.

Edema, or waterlogging, is one of the commonest symptoms of a severe protein deficiency. Actually, this condition stems from a blood disorder, since the extremely delicate balance of water in bloody tissues is chiefly dependent on *blood proteins*. It is the duty of blood proteins to maintain sufficient pressure on the inside of the blood vessel walls to counteract the pressure from the tissues outside the walls. In this way, provided the blood protein is up to normal, the water in blood cannot escape into surrounding tissues and cause the body to become waterlogged. Not so many years ago, this condition was called "dropsy" and was a blood condition that caused untold needless suffering until nutritional science discovered that high-protein diets both prevented and helped clear up this potentially serious ailment.

Cancer, the second of the killer diseases among the older age bracket, has been discussed from a nutritional standpoint in Chapter 7. Exhaustive laboratory studies seem to provide evidence that high-calorie, sugar-and-starch diets nourish the cancerous cells, thereby permitting them to compete with healthy cells, and to gradually reach the final stage when they kill off the healthy cells. The danger of cancer striking in any body, at any age, is too grave to invite it through wrong eating. Be wise now. Replace heavy starch meals with a low-calorie, high-protein diet, and lessen the chances of cancer ever putting its deadly finger on you.

Infection is another of the principal causes, listed by the insurance company pamphlet, that bring death to older persons. Every one of us is ceaselessly exposed to attack by bacteria, viruses and other toxic agents. Yet if you are properly nourished, these lethal bodies seldom get the opportunity to pull off their dirty work. What holds them in check?

Nature provided you with *antibodies*, a first-line defense against infection. These antibodies are formed of protein. *Your resistance to disease germs, and to various other toxins, actually rises or falls according to the amount of high-protein foods you eat.* Dr. Paul R. Cannon of the University of Chicago declared that a high level of resistance to disease can be maintained only on meals containing ample proteins.

Experiments have disclosed that in persons placed on a high-protein diet as many as *100 times* more antibodies show up in the bloodstream within the short period of one week.

If you're not equipped by correct diet to resist infections, then you certainly can't hope to live a long time, or to look and feel younger than your years. Infectious diseases, even if they don't kill you, leave their mark on a body trying to remain youthful.

The fourth of the killer diseases, circulatory disorders, I shall discuss fully under the Sixth Commandment.

SECOND COMMANDMENT—MINERALS WITHOUT FAIL

Minerals rank with protein as the most neglected, haphazardly obtained nutrients in our American diet. And more especially in the diets of persons past forty. One of the "three starvations of later years," spoken of frequently in nutritional reports, is mineral starvation. (The other two "starvations" in older bodies are protein and vitamin B-complex.)

Protein and minerals are so closely linked that to advise you to eat plenty of protein, without stressing the need for equal care in obtaining a full quota of minerals, would be to tell only half the Eat-and-Grow-Younger story.

A report to the National Academy of Sciences by a research team headed by Dr. Cannon emphasizes that the minerals potassium, phosphorus and magnesium are essential in the diet for proper use of all body-building protein foods.

This research team discovered that omitting potassium from the diet could lead to eventual congestive heart failure. Dead tissue developed within the heart muscles.

Six days after potassium was restored to the diet, the body muscles began to rebuild, and the dead tissues in the heart healed.

In other words, with potassium again present, protein could resume its appointed task of repairing and replacing body cells.

Protein and minerals are the chief actors in the nutritional drama, while vitamins play a secondary, although essential, role as *activators,* that is, substances needed to set other substances into action. To neglect any of these three food elements is to wreck the nutritional drama.

Each of the three food elements—protein, minerals, vitamins—has its own specific task in preparing your body for a long, youthful life.

Dr. C. Ward Crampton, noted authority on diseases of older persons, states: "The foremost nutritional defects in the mature and aging are calcium, iron and protein. Seventy-five per cent of the men of sixty suffer a lack of one or more. On the other hand, many suffer dietary excesses, notably carbohydrates and possibly cholesterol."

Calcium is so important an ingredient of your blood that your bloodstream will attempt to maintain its calcium level, even though it has to rob other body parts of their vitally needed calcium. That is why, in many older persons, the bones, robbed of their calcium by the blood, become more fragile, resulting in easily fractured arms, legs and hips.

It is also why calcium-starved heart muscles and brain cells often give up the struggle to maintain normal functioning in bodies that are comparatively young in years.

Your nerves, your heart, your teeth, your brain cells, your blood—all need sufficient calcium to remain healthy, and to function as nature intended.

Commenting that "calcium poverty is one common cause of aging that can be corrected," Dr. Crampton prescribes a grain of calcium lactate for each year of your age, taken in three doses three hours after each meal.

An inexpensive and convenient way to obtain added calcium in the diet is through the use of powdered skim milk. This dry milk provides needed calcium and protein, along with iron, copper, manganese, cobalt and other trace minerals —less the fats which are wisely limited during the later years. (For more on the nutritional values of powdered skim milk see Chapter 11.)

Even though you obtain ample calcium in your diet, quite unknowingly you may be allowing certain foods to rob your body of this vital mineral.

Beet greens and spinach contain oxalic acid which deprives the body of its calcium; but you can eat turnip greens, kale and dandelion greens with full assurance that you are not upsetting the balance of this valuable mineral in your body.

In fact, dandelion greens—that springtime dish of your childhood—have a high calcium and vegetable protein content which make them an excellent spring salad.

Also, don't indulge in cocoa or rhubarb too freely, since both of them have a high oxalic acid content, and by frequent use of these two foods you run the risk of lowering your calcium reserves.

It is Dr. Crampton's belief that a deficiency of *iron* is nearly always present in the "uncared-for person in the higher-age brackets."

He says that the typical person of sixty is anemic, iron-poor and body-poor, unnecessarily so. And this condition is worse in those persons who are following some unwise diet because of "dyspepsia" or "indigestion." Insufficient hydrochloric acid in the gastric secretions is a common cause of iron poverty in the older body. (See Chapter 18.)

Minerals that regulate everything in the human body from "sight to sex" are lacking in a vast acreage of the croplands that spread across our country.

Agricultural scientists are accumulating more and more evidence that a wide variety of human ills are caused by the poor nutrition furnished by foods grown in mineral-starved soils.

Dr. K. Starr Chester, head of a staff of farm researchers, has announced that numerous studies show the soil in nearly every state lacks one or more trace elements—cobalt, copper, zinc, manganese, boron.

All food grown on mineral-poor soil (and the soil on American farms is estimated to have lost from 50 per cent upwards of its mineral contents in the past fifty-five years) is dangerously inadequate in iron, calcium, phosphorus, sodium, potassium, magnesium and sulphur.

For this reason, I cannot say to you with confidence that such-and-such a vegetable or fruit will provide you with this, that or the other mineral. I can tell you that a certain food *should* provide certain minerals. But, strictly speaking, the only way I know of at the present time to give you foolproof advice on minerals is to recommend the use of a reliable mineral concentrate, provided you are in doubt about the mineral content of the foods available to you. The multiple-mineral concentrate is the best way to use a mineral supplement to the diet.

In whatever way you choose to obtain your full daily quota of minerals, for the sake of the restored youthfulness and the long life you so ardently desire, don't neglect these vital food elements. They are minute-to-minute essentials to your health.

THIRD COMMANDMENT—VITAMINS IN
THEIR RIGHTFUL PLACE

The constant need for vitamin-rich food in your diet is an oft-told tale, and one which I shall not repeat here. Yet there are two facts about vitamins which you may not know, and which deserve to be included here.

The first little-known fact about vitamins is that *proteins and vitamins work together*. The chemical agents called *enzymes*, that do the greatest part of the digestive work for your body, are all made of protein (at least those which have been analyzed successfully so far). Certain of these protein enzymes actually take part in your body's use of its vitamins, while certain vitamins affect the body's production of protein enzymes—a sort of "mutual aid society."

In other words, you can't expect the vitamins in your food (or the vitamin supplement you take) to give you all the benefits you expect from them, unless you also provide your body with *ample quantities of protein foods* each day.

Nutritional science has learned that successful vitamin therapy depends upon the presence of adequate high-proteins in the diet. Some biochemists even go so far as to declare that *niacin* (an important member of the vitamin B-complex group) is actually formed from an amino acid (protein) in the first place. Thus, you learn that your *vitamin needs should always begin with a high-protein diet*.

Under ideal conditions, the carefully planned Eat-and-Grow-Younger menus given in Part II should provide you with sufficient vitamins, provided (1) that the greatest care has been exercised in the picking and marketing of the foods before reaching your table, (2) that after arriving in your kitchen, all the foods have been given expert care in preparation and cooking in order not to destroy or waste most of the highly soluble or easily destroyed vitamins, and (3) that all vegetables, fruits and grains have been grown on mineral-rich soil, for it must be remembered that foods grown in mineral-deficient soil may also be poor in vitamins.

Even the trace minerals have a direct effect on the vitamin content of a crop. For example, plants deficient in boron will also contain little vitamin C.

Only when the good earth is mineral-rich can it produce food plants containing all the nutrients vital to the health of the men and animals that feed on them. Much of the meat and poultry that should be a rich source of the various vitamins in the B-complex group, *riboflavin* especially, in reality contain inadequately varied amounts of these food elements, because the animals and fowls were fed on plants and grain which, in turn, were mineral-starved from being grown on depleted soils.

Fruits and vegetables may appear fresh and green in the market, yet be grossly lacking in vitamins, and minerals as well. Nearly half of all farm lands and truck gardens are occupied by tenant farmers who are far more interested in immediate profits than they are in improving the landlords' soil, or in sending to market foods containing all the minerals and vitamins you and I need for maximum health.

Therefore, unless you grow your own fruits and vegetables on organically, *non-chemically* fertilized soil—or can purchase them from farms and gardens containing carefully enriched soil to your certain knowledge—there is every possibility you are not obtaining in your food all the vitamins and minerals needed to keep you looking and feeling young.

It is easy to say "Get your daily vitamins in your foods." The realistic fact is that our foods just do not supply all the vitamins (and minerals) that we should have.

We are living in a most unusual age. Our defense program is geared to high explosives, our production lines are miracles of speed. And our food has "gone modern" to keep pace. It is now being shot out of cannons, super-refined and shaped and coated with highly intriguing artificial preparations. Some of the products have been so highly transformed they are hard to recognize as food.

The case against nutritionally-poor "refined" food—(which has very unrefined manners once it is inside your body)—is growing daily.

Commercial corn meal is one case in point. By the time it reaches your kitchen, it has been largely deprived of its natural vitamin and mineral food values. It has been proved that chickens fed on such refined corn meal die in less than fifty days.

When it has been robbed of its natural vitamins and minerals, food is no longer "food" in the true sense of the word. I wish I could tell you to eat your meat, eggs, dairy products, fruits, vegetables, whole grains, and seed cereals with every assurance that your body would be supplied with sufficient vitamins to keep it healthily youthful—and leave the subject at that. But I cannot.

We who buy our food at the market, or who eat most of our meals away from home, are at the mercy of today's mineral-starved, eroded, artificially fertilized, overcultivated soils—to say nothing of all the vitamin-ignorant cooks.

For that reason, *in addition to good eating,* the safest course is to supplement your Eat-and-Grow-Younger program with a reliably manufactured vitamin-mineral concentrate. There are many good brands available.

Be sure that the vitamin-mineral formula you decide on is really complete. It stands to nutritional reason that the more complete the formula, the more you get for your money—and the better vitamin-mineral insurance you will have. A formula that I personally find thoroughly satisfactory is called Nutri-Time. You might look into it for your own use. It is available in most health-food stores.

Should you take "single" vitamins along with the all-inclusive formula? That depends. Suppose you have developed some deficiency-condition that needs immediate attention. You've seen your doctor and he has advised you to take one or more single vitamins to correct that deficiency. (It might be more vitamin A for night blindness; more vitamin C for spongy, bleeding gums; more vitamin E for heart disorders, and so on.)

But the use of a *single* high-potency vitamin which your doctor recommended is usually for a given period of time— three to six months, depending on individual response. After the specific deficiency has been overcome, it's no longer necessary to use single vitamins in such high potency.

The aim then is to take a vitamin-mineral food supplement that will maintain the body's optimum intake of all vitamins to prevent some future deficiency. And that is where a formula like Nutri-Time can be so helpful to you. You use the complete vitamin-mineral formula every day of your life as a protective food supplement.

Carefully planned meals, plus added vitamins in concentrated form, provide the only way I know of whereby you can make certain that vitamins are "adequate" in your diet. And adequate they must be, if you don't want your Eat-and-Grow-Younger program to bog down at the very start.

FOURTH COMMANDMENT—A MINIMUM OF CARBOHYDRATES

The nutritional folly of gorging yourself on starchy and sweet foods was fully discussed in Chapter 7. But I want to make sure that you do not confuse *natural* carbohydrates with the artificial, devitalized carbohydrates that find their way into American stomachs in such appalling quantities— white breads, cakes, pastries, spaghetti, macaroni, noodles, white rice, processed corn meal, dry cereals (many cooked cereals, too), candies, and carbonated beverages.

A minimum of carbohydrates means: Eliminate *all* those artificial starches which bear small resemblance to the carbohydrates found in natural foods.

Compare the sweetness and flavor of an apple or an orange with that in a piece of candy sweetened with highly refined white sugar crystals, containing absolutely no vitamins or minerals, and colored and flavored with chemicals taken from coal tar.

Compare the flavors and the health benefits of succulent vegetables with that of pure-starch macaroni.

Compare the nutritive sweetness of fruit juices or low-fat milk with that of artificially flavored, colored and carbonated soft drinks.

There is no comparison.

Natural carbohydrates nourish and revitalize your body, since they are sources of minerals, vitamins and some proteins. But all that the highly advertised artificial carbohydrates can do for you is to lead you directly toward a premature old age.

Half your planned campaign to regain your youthful appearance and energy will be won when you throw artificial, devitalized sugars and starches out of your daily eating. Then reward yourself for this commendable step by turning instead to the delicious, health-building sweets I have provided for you in Part II. With these recipes for sweets you can "dissipate," and still not wander from the path of good nutrition.

FIFTH COMMANDMENT—REDUCE WITH REASON

Everyone is pretty well agreed these days that overweight shortens your life—and certainly it prevents your looking and feeling as young as you would desire. Nothing is more aging or more inimical to a youthful appearance than obesity.

Therefore, if you are seriously overweight, begin a sane reducing program at once—for the sake of your health, as well as your youthful appearance. (See Part II for menus planned by calorie count that allow you far more food, and of a better quality, than you ever dreamed would be included in a reducing diet.)

But you must *reduce with reason*.

This means eating high-protein meals. High-protein foods not only stimulate your thyroid gland into producing more of the hormone that keeps the body weight normal but also provide you with the energy and *satisfied* appetite that keep a reducing program from turning into a prolonged torture of weakness and gnawing hunger.

Protein has the power of stimulating greater use of energy by the body. Because of its specific dynamic action *protein yields about 30 per cent more energy* than would be expected from the actual quantity of food eaten. That is, 100 calories of protein food actually yields from 130 to 140 calories of food energy. From this you can readily appreciate that the thrifty, health-wise dieter will spend his calories on protein, *the food that gives him the most energy for the quantity consumed*.

But the overweight person who foolishly invests his day's calories in fad reducing diets—bananas and tomatoes, or rice and pineapple juice, to name but two of the popular reducing regimens—will soon find himself bankrupt, that is, undernourished and under-energized. Further, if he remains too long on one of these lopsided diets, he may actually undermine his health, to say nothing of having a hard time losing more than a few pounds—the hard way.

It has been my experience that the high-protein dieters are actually so well satisfied by their nutritious meals that they yield far less to the temptation of fattening foods than do those dieters who undertake an unwisely planned regimen. Protein foods satisfy the appetite in fewer calorie amounts; that is an added reason why high-protein foods are musts in the diet of the past-forty person who must watch his weight.

A high percentage of all obese persons are also *anemic*. This may come as a surprise to you, since no doubt you've been accustomed to thinking of anemia in the terms of thin, undernourished persons. But you can be *overweight and undernourished* at one and the same time!

Starchy foods, the mealtime mainstay of most obese persons, may satisfy the appetite. But they dull the desire for nourishing high-proteins and mineral-and-vitamin-rich green vegetables and fresh fruits.

The sweets fiend will slight his salad and meat course to settle down in blissful enjoyment over the taste thrills of his rich dessert. Maybe even indulge himself with a second or third helping. And the more starchy foods he eats, the more undernourished and anemic he becomes—and the fatter.

So merely because you may be well-padded with surplus flesh is no guarantee that you are red-blooded and healthy. Usually, the opposite is true.

If you should reduce to safeguard your health, and to look and feel younger, then by all means start doing so immediately. But first make sure that you actually are overweight, since *ideal weight is not emaciation,* as too many of the ladies seem to believe. Then, after you find you really weigh more than is good for your health and your appearance, follow the carefully worked-out reducing regimen provided in Part II.

SIXTH COMMANDMENT—YOUNG ARTERIES ABOVE ALL ELSE

Arteries are seldom mentioned these days without the companion words "hardening" and "cholesterol." A lot of misconception has arisen from half-understood reports issued by physicians and medical laboratories on the need to "limit the diet" to avoid hardening of the arteries (arteriosclerosis), the condition which sometimes leads to a heart seizure or to ruptured blood vessels in the brain.

To clear up some of the potentially harmful misconceptions that have sprung up around "cholesterol and hardening of the arteries," let me explain what cholesterol really is.

Cholesterol is a fat-like substance evidently vital to human life, since it is found in every living cell. It also abounds in the liver, the adrenal glands (in the cortex, or outer layer, of these glands), in the brain and in the nerves. Biochemists are frank to admit that they are still far from understanding very much of the mystery surrounding this fatty substance. Yet it has been noted that cholesterol does have a close biochemical relationship to vitamin D, to the bile acids produced in the liver for digestion of fats, to the hormones secreted by the cortex of the adrenal glands and to the hormones produced by the sex glands of both sexes.

Since cholesterol occurs in such abundance in all living matter, we know that it's essential to the body. We also have established beyond all doubt that the body can manufacture the cholesterol it needs. Further, we know that under *normal conditions* excess, unwanted amounts of this fatty substance can be destroyed in the body.

But the most important thing for you to remember about cholesterol is this: *The consumption of heavy starches causes deposits of cholesterol to form in the body, mainly in the arteries.*

Laboratory animals—dogs and rabbits—were taken off their natural diets of meats and green, leafy foods. Instead they were fed on the ordinary human diet containing quantities of artificial starches, plus fatty foods.

Within an astonishingly short time, the arteries of these starch-and-fat fed animals were found to have become "hardened," that is, deposits of cholesterol had piled up in the arteries, overlaid with deposits of calcium sent by the blood in an attempt to "heal" the damaged artery.

For that is exactly what happens to a hardened artery—it becomes brittle and less flexible because of the deposits of cholesterol and calcium that keep piling up on the inner arterial wall. Yet when their natural diets were restored to these laboratory animals, their arteries stopped "hardening." Moreover, it was noted that some of the cholesterol and calcium deposits on their arterial walls were being reabsorbed.

Dr. Daniel C. Munro, one of the pioneers in the low-starch, high-protein diet, reports he personally has observed that dogs—meat-eaters by nature—will develop hardening of the arteries and arthritis after starchy foods are given them in considerable quantities.

Today, some medical scientists place the blame for too much cholesterol in the blood on foods that actually are valuable sources of nutrition—egg yolk, liver, gland meats and vegetable oils. Diets are being prescribed that greatly restrict the use of these excellent foods.

Also prohibited are pork, pies, rich cakes, cookies and all fried foods—none of which, of course, should be given a place in *any* diet.

Nothing, however, seems to be said about white bread, devitalized cereals, white rice, macaroni and similar pure-starch items.

Now let's check into the practical wisdom of these "low-fat" diets currently being prescribed indiscriminately for persons suspected of having "hardened" arteries.

Fats, the same as carbohydrates, are used by the body to supply heat and energy. Right at the start, we begin to realize that the average American diet is top-heavy with two food elements—fats and carbohydrates—both with the same nutritional function, that of providing heat and energy.

Carbohydrates, when too plentiful in the diet, usurp the natural function of the fat foods, thereby allowing the fats to be deposited instead of being *burned* for energy. The fats you eat must be used for energy; otherwise they are "hoarded" in the tissues and in the *arteries*.

It's wrong to give fats a "black eye." Our bodies need fats. But there are "good" fats as well as "bad" fats. It is the latter you must watch—*particularly* if you are at all concerned about hardening of the arteries and heart disease.

In the health-interest of your heart and arteries, I urge you to eliminate ALL *processed* fats from your diet.

How can this be done?

First of all, cross off your list anything that has been "hydrogenated." The label will tell you. Solid shortenings are hydrogenated. So is margarine. The average commercial peanut butter is no exception.

Many factory-made foods contain hydrogenated fats. This means crackers, prepared "mixes," noodles, roasted and salted nuts, popcorn. It means any food fried in deep fat—potato chips, french fries, doughnuts.

The fats and oils you can substitute for these are the so-called *highly unsaturated* salad oils (safflower oil, sunflower oil, sesame oil, soybean oil, corn oil—are among the best).

Even though you may on occasion "go overboard" in the use of animal fats like butter and cream, among others, the important point to keep in mind as far as cholesterol deposits are concerned, is that the *unsaturated* vegetable oils are to be the dominant fats in your diet.

It is vital to keep in mind that a certain amount of the right kind of food fat is essential for supplying a proper amount of the body fat that protects us from shock, checks our loss of heat by radiation and promotes the mobility of our bodies.

It is only when fats are *eaten to excess,* or when they are *combined with high-carbohydrate meals,* that they pile up in all those unwanted and dangerous places—around the waist, in the liver, around the heart and on the inner walls of the arteries.

It's not difficult to understand that when you eat a high-starch meal which also includes a quantity of fat, you are *overfueling* your body.

If you've ever flooded the carburetor in your car with too much gasoline, or choked out the fire in your furnace by piling on too much coal, you can readily understand that overfueling is something to be avoided. Unburned gasoline floods out the carburetor in your car, unburned coal clogs up the grate in your furnace and *unburned fats* pile up on the walls of your arteries.

By eliminating all high-starch foods you can force your body to burn its fat deposits instead of keeping it refueled each day.

When the body receives no carbohydrates, the "goldbricking" fats are called out of their hiding place in the arteries and put to work. Since there are no sugars and starches to provide energy, the stored deposits of fat in the arteries—in the tissues, as well—are mustered into the bloodstream to supply the body with heat and energy.

Strangely enough, the amount of cholesterol found in the

blood of persons known to have severely damaged arteries is quite *low*. The only apparent explanation for this is that when cholesterol from our food is being properly utilized, it circulates freely in the bloodstream to the points of the body requiring it. But when carbohydrate foods are continually "subbing" for cholesterol, this fat sneaks off to pile up on the artery walls.

Isn't it more logical to eliminate the artificial, high-starch foods in the diet—foods that we can live very nicely without and be far healthier for the omitting—than to take away certain valuable foods like eggs, cheese, liver and gland meats, and *unsaturated* vegetable oils which are rich sources of urgently needed vitamins and minerals? I'm encouraged to see that some of our more conservative medical men aren't quite ready to accept the theory that hardening of the arteries can be either cured or prevented merely by omitting these fat-containing foods from the diet.

Dr. Munro cites the case of a man in his seventies, a liberal carbohydrate-eater, who suffered an attack of coronary thrombosis (a heart block caused by hardened arteries). This diagnosis was confirmed by an electrocardiogram read by leading heart specialists. The patient was then placed on a high-protein, low-carbohydrate diet which he followed to the letter. Two years later—when normally he would have expected to become a total invalid, if not deceased, because of his serious heart condition—an electrocardiogram showed *no sign of thrombosis*. And seven years later he was still free of this highly dangerous heart condition.

The only explanation of this almost phenomenal betterment in an extremely serious arterial condition is that the low-carbohydrate diet forced his body to clear out the fat deposits in his more-than-seventy-year-old arteries to provide him with heat and energy, replacing the denied high-carbohydrates as energizers. Meanwhile, the high-protein foods in his diet set about immediately repairing the damage previously inflicted on the arterial walls by the calcium and fat deposits.

I have not the slightest hesitancy in declaring that it's my belief that this patient would not have shown this astonishing recovery if he had been put on a diet restricting "eggs, cheese, glandular meats and vegetable oils," and allowing him unrestricted carbohydrates.

My advice to you on "eating to keep your arteries young" would be only half complete if I were to neglect reporting the encouraging results being obtained in hundreds of cases of hardened arteries treated with *choline* and *inositol*—two members of the well-known vitamin B-complex family.

(Dr. Dutchess reported that, in addition to choline and inositol, the B-vitamin *pyridoxine* and a food protein called *methionine*—one of the 10 essential amino acids described in Chapter 5—are necessary in the diet to help prevent cholesterol from becoming lazy and settling down in the arteries.)

Choline, a fat-dissolving agent, is a wonderful aid in promoting normal distribution of food fat throughout the body in the proper storage places provided for fat (under the skin is one such place). In other words, choline helps food fats to find their normal resting places in the body, thereby preventing the stockpiling of fat in undesirable spots, notably in hardening arteries and in a fat-clogged liver.

Choline, inositol and *pyridoxine*, as members of the vitamin B-complex group, are found in most high-protein foods—lean beef and lamb, organ meats (liver, kidney, heart, brains, sweetbreads), eggs, cheese, seed cereals—and in whole grains.

A choline, inositol and pyridoxine deficiency results mainly from a diet low in protein, and high in fats and carbohydrates. This describes the high-carbohydrate, artificial, devitalized food diets that comprise more than 80 per cent of all American meals.

If you want to avoid the *circulatory disorders* which rank among the chief killers past the age of forty, then my earnest plea to you is this: *Starting with your next meal, put yourself for life on a high-protein, low-starch diet.*

And, above all, don't be panicked by half-understood published reports of experiments on arteriosclerosis into omitting certain high-protein foods which are among your richest sources of the fat-controlling B-vitamins, choline, inositol and pyridoxine. If for any valid reason you cannot consistently follow a high-protein diet, then I urge you to obtain supplemental daily amounts of choline, inositol and pyridoxine. Otherwise, your intake of these fat-controlling B-vitamins is likely to be inadequate to prevent the accumulation of cholesterol on the arterial walls.

Lecithin granules—(obtainable at all health food stores)—will provide you with an extremely reliable and potent source of choline and inositol. The vitamin-mineral supplement you should use anyway will, if it is a good formula, take care of any extra needs you may have for pyridoxine.

Incidentally, choline is also found in the seeds of an herb known as fenugreek, a member of the legume family. As an added precaution against the stockpiling of fats in the liver and arteries, you might consider getting acquainted with this pleasant-tasting herb made into a mealtime or between-meal tea.

So now you have been given the *Six Commandments For A Long, "Young" Life*. Within them lies the nucleus of all dietary truth. They are the keystone of all your efforts to become a trim, radiant person, glowing with health and energy.

Chapter 10

SEEDS HOLD THE GERM OF LIFE

MODERN diets ignore the axiom that seeds hold the germ of life. Too often overlooked is the fact that nature has placed in seed foods the concentrated essence of all nutrition in order to provide nourishment for the sprouting plant.

Only one part of any plant is outstandingly rich in protein and that is the seed. Proteins are centered in the seeds of a plant, so that the new life may receive ample nourishment for normal growth.

Little by little, modern nutritional science is inclining to the belief that *whole* seed cereals (I stress "whole" because of the health-blind custom of milling most of the food value out of our cereals) can supply for your diet a now missing *something* that formerly was there when life and eating habits were much closer to the primitive.

In fact, several biochemists have told me it's their private opinion that only when we regain that missing "something" in our diets which the primitive peoples enjoyed will we find the preventive for many of our deficiency and wasting diseases.

Seed foods have always formed a large portion of the instinctive diet followed by primitive peoples. Yet how many times this past year has *your* table been graced with millet, steel-cut oats, whole unbolted cornmeal, raw wheat germ, sesame seed or sunflower seed?

Have your pancakes and muffins been made with all-starch white flower or devitalized corn meal—or with whole wheat flour and millet meal?

Does your cereal bowl at breakfast contain a no-food-value, devitalized dry cereal—or does it contain steel-cut oats, or millet meal mush?

Unless you are one of the disturbingly small minority in this country who recognizes the stay-young values in seed cereals, your pancakes were made with 100 per cent-starch white flour, your muffins with devitalized corn meal, your cereal bowl contained a patented dry cereal.

And yet you wonder why your hair turns gray, muscles grow flabby, figure becomes lumpy, teeth decay, eyesight grows poorer, sexual powers disappear prematurely and nerves act like Mexican jumping beans.

Let me introduce you to several of the new-old seed cereals about which you probably know very little. They merit a place in every diet, for they will help build a body that is firm and lithe—*a young body*.

MILLET

Millet is the first of the seed cereals that should be on your table regularly.

Perhaps best known as poultry and animal feed, millet has been one of the principal grains of Eastern Europe, Africa, Siberia and China for centuries. Five hundred years before the beginning of the modern Christian era, the Greek philosopher Pythagoras praised the high nutritive value of millet, and advised his followers (all vegetarians) to adopt millet as the mainstay of their diets.

Contrary to popular belief, millet and not rice is the basic food of most Chinese in their native country. Only the small-statured, less robust Southern Chinese subsist on rice. The tall, sturdy, vigorous Northern Chinese have used millet as their principal food for many centuries.

We Americans will adopt a certain plant from other continents, but for our livestock, not for our own bodies. Our appetites tend to spurn the wholesome, health-giving, youth-protective natural foods in favor of widely advertised artificial foods that make old men and women of us in our prime.

One Saturday morning, while driving to the West Coast, I stopped in a small Iowa town located in the heart of a rich farming section, and parked in front of the local grocery store. The street was lined with farmers' trucks and autos while the families went about their weekly shopping.

Before long the family in the car next to mine returned, loaded down with their purchases—the father carrying a sack labeled "Whole Millet, Chicken Feed, Mineral-and-Protein Rich, For Laying Stock"; the children alternately lapping on ice cream cones or munching on candy bars; and the mother carrying a box of canned goods topped by two loaves of baker's white bread (even sliced for her) and a cellophane package of dried noodles. What a travesty on good nutrition!

The only real nourishment in all their purchases—the whole

millet—was going to their chickens, while the devitalized white-flour bread and noodles were supposed to "nourish" the hard-working farmer and farm wife and their growing children. Watching them as they drove away, I could have wept for the long-life days when a farmer took his own grain to the mill to be ground *whole,* then returned it to the barrel in the pantry; and the farm wife made her own bread and noodles from the whole grain flour.

Millet is one of the oldest and most nutritious foods known to man. It is a balanced grain, rich in high-grade protein, minerals, vitamins and *lecithin* (the same tasty substance found in egg yolk, and containing valuable *choline.*)

Laboratory investigations have revealed that few foods are digested with greater ease than millet. It does not ferment in the stomach, causing digestive and intestinal distress, as do foods made from white flour and other devitalized grains.

After World War I, millions of Russian peasants in White Russia faced starvation. In desperation, they ate the millet which had been put away for the chickens they no longer had. And what happened? Not only did these peasants survive the long period of famine, but they soon discovered they were enjoying better health than they had ever known while consuming their former varied diets.

One of the peasants, who had suffered from stomach ulcers for fifteen years, found that his ulcers disappeared in six months on his forced diet of nothing but millet.

Dr. John Harvey Kellogg declared that millet is the only cereal capable of supporting human life when used as the sole item in the diet. Of course, no one wants to live exclusively on millet—unless forced to do so as were those desperate Russian peasants. But if worse came to worst, scientists are convinced that you could live on a diet of nothing but millet, and not only survive, but become even healthier and more vigorous than you ever were.

This is a fact which I believe should be more widely utilized by dietitians and homemakers during times of meat scarcities and meat rationing. During meat rationing, home economists promoted, as meat substitutes, rice, macaroni, spaghetti and noodle dishes.

Starch is never a safe substitute for protein.

The only foods which should ever appear in the menu as an honest substitute for a meat dish are eggs, cheese, milk and high-protein seed cereals. By adding extra amounts of dry skim milk (a rich source of protein) to these truly protein meat substitutes, a meatless diet may be prevented from falling far below a safe daily minimum of 100 to 150 grams of protein.

Now don't get the idea that I'm recommending that you do away with meat in your diet, and substitute millet. Meat is an unexcelled, hard-to-replace food, but there are thousands of persons living on incomes that won't permit their purchasing meat every day in the week. For that reason, I believe that more recognition should be given to millet as a nutritionally safe, low-cost, easily digestible meat substitute.

Millet for human use is available at all health-food stores. The variety sold in feed or bird stores is not fit for human consumption, since the hard, outer coat has not been removed. This makes it impossible to cook.

For that reason, when buying millet seed, it is wise to be sure to get the "hulled" variety. Millet is also available ground into a meal, which can be used in precisely the same way corn meal is used.

PREPARING MILLET PORRIDGE

In preparing millet porridge—(using either the "hulled" seed or the ground meal)—one cup of millet to four cups of liquid is about right. Heat the liquid—which may be water, milk, or half-water-half-milk—until it bubbles. Add the millet slowly, stirring constantly to prevent scorching or sticking. Serve with honey for a delicious breakfast treat!

Millet is a seed cereal which is both satisfying and easily digestible. It merits a place in every diet, for gradually it will take away your desire for white breads and rich pastries.

And after you've succeeded in eliminating all artificial, pure-starch, youth-destroying foods from your diet, your body will show its gratitude by losing that bloated, flabby look which puts the years on you along with the pounds.

SUNFLOWER SEEDS

Sunflower seeds are another highly nutritious seed food that we can supply generously to our parrots and our chickens, yet neglect to utilize in raising the standards of our under-par human diets.

Back in the days of the czars, every Russian soldier out in the campaign field was given what was called his daily "iron ration"—a two-pound bag of sunflower seeds. Because the army away from its supply bases was sometimes forced to live exclusively on these seeds, the officers furnished their men with this tasty, lightweight food knowing that it gave them all the nourishment needed to keep them in good condition.

(Besides the protein, vitamins and other minerals, two pounds of sunflower seeds contain about 21 milligrams of *iron*. The average grown man requires at least 12 milligrams of iron each day for optimum health, while the average woman needs a minimum of 15 milligrams. From these figures it's easy to understand that the Russian soldier in those days must have been a red-blooded fellow.)

The Russians, Turks and Arabs living near the Black Sea and in Asia Minor chew sunflower seeds as Americans chew gum. Every Russian home in that region has a bowlful of sunflower seeds to be dipped into at all times.

Within the last several years, various scientists over the country have made studies to ascertain the nutritional values of the sunflower seed. An experiment conducted to compare sunflower seeds with wheat germ, corn germ and soybeans obtained these results:

Sunflower seeds are the best vegetable source of niacin, the "courage" vitamin. Niacin is so lacking in modern diets that 100,000 cases of pellagra—the disease caused by its deficiency—occur each year.

Niacin helps to overcome suspicion, hostility, and depression, the very ills from which cocktail sippers might seek relief. The most courageous people, when they become pellagrins, turn cowardly, apprehensive, suspicious, and confused.

Further investigations revealed that sunflower seeds contain about *60 percent more pantothenic acid* (likewise a member of the B-vitamin family, and sometimes known as the "anti-gray hair vitamin") than soybean meal; and considerably more pantothenic acid than either corn germ or wheat germ.

It was also learned that sunflower seeds top the list of all vegetable concentrates, containing *55.4 per cent high-grade protein*.

The report concluded: "Sunflower seeds are unusually rich in bone-forming *calcium*. It is an excellent source of *thiamine*, or vitamin B-1."

We have since discovered that sunflower seeds are regular storehouses for the minerals *silicon, magnesium, fluorine* and *phosphorus*, in addition to their particularly generous amounts of *calcium* and *iron*.

Because of the flower's close affinity to the sun, sunflower seeds are an extremely rich source of *vitamin D*, being one of the very few plants containing this "sunshine vitamin."

Sunflower seeds may enter your diet in several ways.

The hulled seeds make a delicious confection, with a flavor

far superior, in my opinion, to peanuts. Sunflower seeds, hulled and sometimes toasted, have been a delicacy in the Orient and in Slavic countries for many centuries.

The vegetarians who have tried "meat loaf" made of ground sunflower seeds declare it to be far superior in both flavor and nourishment to any other substitute they have found. Sunflower seeds contain a protein that approaches meat protein in taste and smell. The meal made from sunflower seeds mixes well with other flours, and bakes quickly. It is delicious, too, when used for thickening soups, gravies and sauces.

Sunflower seeds should be an essential in every vegetarian diet, as well as in the diets of those persons who are seeking economical, easily digested, youth-protecting proteins. The protein content of sunflower seeds is better balanced and more digestible than that of soybeans.

If you hear scoffers maintain that sunflower seeds are for the birds, remember that birds are pretty active creatures. It is no surprise to me when enthusiastic reports keep coming in from persons who have adopted sunflower seeds as a regular item in their diets.

Especially interesting is the almost unanimous praise for sunflower seeds as a food that remedies bleeding gums, and slows down tooth decay. Of course, the explanation for this is the unusually high content of the vitamins A and D, and the minerals, calcium, phosphorus, silicon and fluorine, all of them nutrients directly concerned with the health of teeth and gums.

The calcium of raw sunflower seeds is easily assimilated by the human body. This may be one reason why eating sunflower seeds was believed by our grandparents to cure rheumatism. Although no extensive research has been done on this belief as yet, still some of you who suffer from this painful ailment may wish to do some experimenting on your own. About a small handful of hulled seeds is the average daily amount that could be effective.

J. I. Rodale, one of the country's most tireless crusaders for better nutrition, noticed that after eating sunflower seeds for about a month he could walk down a snow-covered road in the bright sunlight without suffering the eyestrain which the dazzling glare had formerly caused.

He noticed, also, that he no longer was troubled with bleeding gums after introducing sunflower seeds into his daily diet. He was further pleased to note that his skin seemed to be getting smoother. Nutritional science has proved that calcium and vitamin A—both of them generously present in sunflower seeds—are an essential in the diet of a person who desires a healthy skin.

Silicon, provided by sunflower seeds in unusually large quantities, enters into the composition of your hair, nails, nerves, blood, albumin and teeth (aided in this last by *fluorine*). Laboratory research has discovered that a deficiency of silicon—a trace mineral—in the diet leads to loss of hair and early decay of teeth, as well as to a greatly lowered resistance to infection.

From what I've told you about sunflower seeds, you should need no urging to add to your diet this food which contains more *riboflavin* than wheat germ, and is an all-around better source of the *B-vitamins* and of *high-grade protein* than any other grain.

The sunflower seed has often been described as "a little sunlamp in your digestive system" which is beneficial to eyesight, complexion, fingernails and acts as a curb on high blood pressure and jumpy nerves.

With so many points in its favor—you'll be giving your health a real nutritional boost by eating a handful or more of these seeds each day. Have them as a snack, like peanuts; sprinkle on fruit salads; mix into scrambled eggs—you'll discover many uses for yourself once you become acquainted with this truly wonder food.

And *don't* try to buy sunflower seeds in bird stores! They are now available, *shelled* (hulled) and *ready to eat,* in health food stores. Considering their nutritional values, sunflower seeds are remarkably reasonable in price.

SESAME SEEDS

You probably know *sesame seeds* as the flat, light-colored seeds which are sometimes used by bakers to sprinkle over loaves of Vienna bread. Until recently this seed was not believed to have any special nutritional value. But early in 1924 an American scientist began an exhaustive study on the nutritional values of sesame seeds, at the same time using these seeds as the exclusive source of protein and fat in his diet. As a result of these studies, and his own personal experimentation, he found that the protein and fat in sesame seeds are unusually easy to digest. This fact makes sesame seeds of special value in the diets of invalids and persons with weak digestive organs.

Sesame seeds, together with millet and sunflower seeds, contain more *lecithin* than the soybean. Lecithin is a phosphorized fat (a compound of phosphorus, fat and nitrogen) which is an important ingredient of the tissues in your nerves, brain and endocrine glands. Your nervous system, for instance, uses lecithin to aid in generating nerve electricity. When your nerves are plentifully supplied with lecithin, your body abounds in nervous energy; and when the supply of lecithin gets low, as it does at the end of the day, your nerve energy decreases, and you say you are "tired and sleepy." A serious deficiency of lecithin in the diet can bring on a nerve exhaustion that is characterized by a chronic fatigue which rest does not alleviate.

Lecithin is also important for your brain, since your "organ of thinking" contains approximately 28 per cent of this substance, that is, provided you are sane. The brains of persons suffering from serious mental illnesses contain less than half this amount of lecithin.

Sesame seeds are known also to contain an important amount of calcium, phosphorus, iron and trace minerals, in addition to their high content of thiamine and the other members of the vitamin B-complex family.

Introduced into your diet, in conjunction with millet and sunflower seeds, sesame seeds can provide an additional seed cereal of high nutritional value. In addition to sprinkling these seeds generously on home-baked breads and cookies (made from whole grain flour, of course), sesame seeds may also be made into a meal by crushing slightly toasted seeds under a rolling pin. This meal may then be sprinkled over salads and hot cereals, mixed with fresh or cooked vegetables for added seasoning, added to soups or combined with other seed meals for something different in the way of a taste delight.

And when it comes to confections, if you've never eaten sesame candy or sesame cookies, you don't know what you've been missing. The Greeks, traditionally famous cooks, make liberal use of sesame seeds in their pastries and confections. I have never tasted anything more delightful than a Greek confection, called "baklava," made principally of sesame seeds and honey. Included in Part II are a number of recipes using sesame seeds. White-sugar and white-flour confections and cookies will add unwelcome years and pounds to your face and figure. But dainties made from whole grains, natural sweeteners and sesame seeds will delight your taste buds at the same time they provide added food values for your planned diet.

Chapter 11

BEST MILKS FOR HUMANS

MILK, man's first and oldest beverage, has taken on a new form that puts it in the front ranks of *concentrated* protective foods. I refer to *dry skim milk*—an inexpensive, readily digested, high-protein food that is handy to use and short on calories.

Liquid milk is dried by being sprayed into compressed air, and the milk solids come out with the fine, smooth texture of face powder. The color is beautifully white with a faint greenish cast caused by the *high-concentration of riboflavin*. The flavor of the new dry skim milk is mild and delicate, and its faint smell resembles that of sweet dried coconut.

I must confess to taking a few liberties with history when I say that dried milk is "new." Actually, long before the birth of Christ the ancient Egyptians prepared a concentrated milk by drying it in the sun.

And the sturdy Mongol horsemen who made up the invading armies of the conqueror Genghis Khan were supplied with sun-dried milk as a concentrated marching ration that would assure them the full nourishment necessary for their strenuous campaigns.

So we're a few centuries late in learning that dried milk is a wonderfully concentrated food.

If everyone in this country were to use this economical food in their daily diet, it could overcome the widespread deficiencies of protein, calcium and riboflavin which afflict thousands upon thousands of persons, causing them to fall ready victims to aging diseases.

Did you know that the addition of even so little as a tablespoonful of powdered skim milk to your daily servings of food would be a worthwhile contribution to your Eat-and-Grow-Younger program?

Did you know that less than one-half cup of powdered skim milk contains all the nutrients found in a quart of fresh skim milk?

Did you know that powdered skim milk contributes far more food value than whole fresh milk because it is so highly concentrated?

Did you know that powdered skim milk is tolerated by persons who find whole fresh milk hard to digest?

Did you know that the highly concentrated amounts of protein, calcium and riboflavin in dry skim milk can help prolong your "prime of life," and aid you in retaining a sexual youthfulness?

Did you know that there are no nutritional values in yogurt over ordinary buttermilk or sour milk? If you like yogurt for its distinctive taste, then by all means use it, for it's a good milk product. But ordinary buttermilk or soured fresh milk will give you almost the same nutritional benefits, particularly lactic acid.

Also, dry skim milk made into a liquid, with lemon juice added to sour it, makes a sour milk that is good to drink and excellent for cooking.

These *milk facts* should be known to everybody, since milk is one food about which much myth and misconception has been built up throughout years of propagandizing by the dairy industry.

Milk, we have been told repeatedly for decades, is a "perfect food," and a "complete food." Like much other propagandizing, these statements are but half-truths. Sweet milk is not a "perfect food" for anyone who cannot digest it properly.

Nor is sweet milk a perfect food when taken at mealtime by persons whose digestive juices are not acid enough to properly digest the protein foods eaten.

Because sweet milk has an alkaline reaction in the stomach, when taken by the glassful at mealtime it tends to counteract the natural acidity of the hydrochloric acid in our digestive juices.

Many persons who had thought they suffered from "chronic dyspepsia" have discovered that their symptoms vanished completely after they ceased drinking sweet milk with their meals. If you like the flavor of fresh milk—and it does not lie in your stomach like a handful of putty—then by all means enjoy it, but *between meals*, and never at mealtime, especially if you have long since celebrated your thirtieth birthday.

Buttermilk as a mealtime beverage is quite a different matter, because its high lactic acid content actually promotes the digestion of proteins and iron-containing foods.

If you'll only stop to think for a minute, you'll realize that nature provided sweet milk for the suckling young animal, unable as yet to masticate solid foods. Nowhere in nature do you find any animal, except man, mixing fresh sweet milk with solid protein foods.

Another mistaken belief popularly held about fresh milk is that the "richer the milk, the better." Nothing could be farther from the truth. The protein, minerals and vitamin B-complex (riboflavin and thiamine mainly) are all contained in the *skim milk*, not in the cream.

Many mothers, for instance, make the mistake of purchasing the richest milk they can find for their children. Yet, instead of gaining in weight and health, their children actually lose weight and have little appetite. The reason for this is that the cream in the rich milk satisfies their appetites too quickly, taking away the desire for larger quantities of other foods containing richer sources of protein, minerals and vitamins. If the children were given skim milk, not only would they drink more of it, but they would eat more heartily of the protective foods. The same holds true for any age.

In many persons the undigested fat in *too rich milk* combines with calcium, thereby preventing this vital mineral from reaching the bloodstream. When this happens, a serious calcium deficiency, with all its aging discomforts and ailments, is likely to result—despite the most earnest of efforts to "drink plenty of milk for calcium."

And, to make matters worse, the combination of fat-and-calcium forms a sort of hard soap in the intestines, causing a hard-to-overcome type of constipation. Perhaps you are one of the many persons who find rich *whole* milk "binding." If so, that is the explanation.

Regardless of whether or not your weight is normal, *dry skim milk is the best sweet milk for you*.

If you want to gain weight, dry skim milk, used liberally, will provide extra amounts of the protein, minerals and vitamins, lack of which probably caused you to be underweight in the first place.

If, on the other hand, overweight is your problem, and yours should be a reducing diet, then dry skim milk is equally good. Liberal amounts of this powdered skim milk can be used without making your calorie count jump up like the thermometer on a hot day. This milk can be incorporated into your reducing menu in a number of flavorful and appetite-satisfying ways.

Moreover, the highly concentrated protein in this type of milk is a valuable aid to a high-protein reducing diet, since the more protein you eat (without adding calories) the more quickly your sluggish thyroid gland can be prodded into taking over and bringing your body weight back to normal.

Then again you may not like the taste of either sweet milk or buttermilk well enough to drink it. If so, dry skim milk makes it possible for you to obtain all the health-protective values in this protein food without offending your sense of taste.

Incorporate at least one-half cup of the milk powder into your food each day, and you'll get all the benefits of a quart of fresh liquid milk. (The menus in Part II do this "incorporating" for you.)

Right now powdered skim milk is the biggest food bargain of all. You can slice your milk bill to a third with powdered skim milk as well as supplementing your diet with the valuable proteins and vitamins and minerals found in this wonderful food.

If you wish to economize and simplify your marketing, you may omit buying fresh milk altogether, and stock your cupboard with the inexpensive, long-keeping dry skim milk powder, to be made up into liquid milk with a few flips of the eggbeater or wire whisk by merely adding it to cold water. And this *reconstructed* liquid milk that you yourself make from skim milk powder can be as diluted or as concentrated as you wish.

From the standpoint of economy and convenience alone, housewives tell me they would not be without dry skim milk after once using it. Yet economy and convenience are but two of the advantages that all health-conscious persons have gained by the advent of this new dry skim milk.

For instance, a tablespoonful of skim milk powder thoroughly mixed into the beaten egg makes wonderful scrambled eggs for breakfast, an excellent high-protein dish with which to start off the day.

At lunch, dry skim milk can be added to soups or to the egg sauce served over vegetables such as asparagus or cauliflower.

Whole-grain bread, made with liberal amounts of powdered skim milk sifted in with the flour, in addition to the normal amount of liquid called for in the recipe, makes a richer, more high-protein bread than ordinarily would be produced.

At dinner, the fruit pudding or egg custard served for dessert should contain a tablespoonful or more of dry skim milk in addition to the liquid milk specified in the recipe.

I don't wish to bore you with statistics. Yet there are certain briefly worded facts about dry skim milk which you should know to better appreciate the necessity for adding this youth-protecting food to your Eat-and-Grow-Younger diet.

So concentrated is dry skim milk that it contains *eleven times* more high-grade protein, minerals, B-vitamins and lactose than fresh whole milk. This means that eleven pounds of fresh milk are used to prepare 1 pound of dry skim milk.

Powdered skim milk is 36.5 per cent protein, as compared to 19.7 per cent protein found in an equal weight of lean beef. So concentrated is this milk powder that when you use it you are providing your body with a food that is more than one-third pure protein of the type classed as complete by biochemists. *In its powdered form,* less than two cups of dry skim milk yields 200 grams of protein—a safe margin over the recommended daily minimum protein requirement of 100 to 150 grams for adults. You can begin to see now why I have added dry skim milk so liberally to the foods in your Eat-and-Grow-Younger menus in Part II. Where else could you get so much concentrated pure protein at so low a cost?

For about 30 cents a day you can furnish 60 per cent of your family's daily protein allowance—four cups of skim milk powder for a family of four. Compare this with getting an equivalent amount of complete protein from other sources. Your savings can be as high as $400 a year.

You can fortify your fresh milk to make it contain 62 per cent more protein by adding one-half cup of powdered skim milk and shaking it.

If you want an extra-juicy, extra-plump, and extra-rich broiled hamburger soon, just add a couple of tablespoons of skim milk powder to the mixture.

An analysis of skim milk powder shows it to be approximately 8 per cent minerals. This is a remarkably high concentration of minerals, since most foods contain less than 1 per cent.

All the important minerals necessary for human health are found in dry skim milk. It is especially rich in calcium and phosphorus. In fact, it is recognized as a richer source of calcium than any other natural food. Three-quarters of a cup of dry skim milk will supply more than your normal daily need for calcium, and about two-thirds of your phosphorus requirements for a day.

Potassium is another essential food mineral generously present in dry skim milk. In fact, the high calcium-phosphorus-potassium concentration in dry skim milk makes it a wonderful nerve, brain and heart re-conditioner for the past-forty body. When combined with phosphorus, potassium helps keep your nervous system strong enough to withstand the tenseness which so often afflicts men and women alike immediately before, during and after their climacteric. Milk, not alcohol or tobacco, will calm your nerves and take away that tenseness which frequently leads to neurotic symptoms—sure signs of age anywhere along the calendar.

Potassium, in combination with calcium, is vital to the youthful action of the older heart. Calcium salts contract the heart muscles, while the potassium salts act to relax them. It is this continual interchange of equalized contraction and relaxation that enables your heart to keep on beating normally, sending out an uninterrupted supply of life-sustaining blood to every cell in your body.

Except for iron and copper (and it does contain small completely usable amounts of these two minerals), dry skim milk is rich in all the important minerals recognized at this time as essential to your health. In addition to those already mentioned, this new powdered milk contains sulphur, chlorine, sodium, magnesium, manganese, iodine, cobalt and zinc.

Dry skim milk is also a particularly rich source of the youth-promoting vitamins in the B-complex group—thiamine, riboflavin, choline, inositol, niacin, pyridoxine, pantothenic acid, para-aminobenzoic acid, biotin, folic acid and vitamin B-12.

More than merely "containing" these B-vitamins, dry skim milk provides them in a *natural balance,* along with its proteins, minerals and carbohydrates. The closer you can stay to a *natural* concentrated food (or to a scientifically combined diet supplement), the more likely you are to obtain a food with all its nutrients in balance.

As mentioned earlier, dry skim milk is one of the most concentrated sources of *riboflavin* yet discovered. I won't go into detail here on all the ways in which riboflavin helps you to feel and look younger. The riboflavin story is fully told in Chapters 13 and 14. But I will warn you right here that if you are not getting enough riboflavin in your everyday diet—and few adult persons do—then you might as well reconcile yourself to feeling and looking much older than you are because, in doing nothing to correct this riboflavin deficiency, you are laying your entire body open to a general speeding up in the aging process.

The age-fighting thiamine, which your nervous system requires in increasingly large amounts after your fortieth birthday, is also present in dry skim milk. One cupful of powdered skim milk will supply more than 25 per cent of your daily requirement for this important B-vitamin. Like riboflavin, thiamine is imperative to a mind and body that stands the years well.

If millet meal is not available to you at this time, you may still provide your body with this age-fighting vitamin by cooking your breakfast corn meal mush, oatmeal or any other whole-grain cooked cereal in liquefied dry skim milk. Then add a balanced vitamin concentrate, containing thiamine, to your daily health program.

Running quickly down the list of the other B-vitamins found in dry skim milk, there is *pyridoxine,* necessary, among other functions, to aid in keeping your nerves young; *pantothenic acid* which, when seriously lacking in the diet, brings on these alarming signs of age: gastro-intestinal lesions, withered testicles, disordered adrenal glands, fatty deposits in the liver and kidneys and gray thinning hair; *choline* and *inositol* which are now recognized as valuable in helping curb hardening of the arteries (see Chapter 9) which causes more deaths among the past-forty group than any other disease; *para-aminobenzoic acid,* now believed to be the real anti-gray hair factor in the B-complex group; *biotin,* vital to complete nutrition of your body; *folic acid* and *vitamin B-12* known to be specifics in the treatment or prevention of anemia.

Although dry skim milk does not contain an appreciable amount of *niacin,* it does provide *tryptophane,* the amino acid from which your body can manufacture its own niacin.

Dry skim milk is 52 per cent carbohydrate. But don't jump to conclusions that I've been advocating a high-carbohydrate food in this chapter, after having denounced high-starch foods earlier in the book. Let me explain—the carbohydrate in dry skim milk is *lactose,* commonly known as "milk sugar."

No ordinary carbohydrate is lactose. While other carbohydrates, such as those found in white flour, white sugar, white rice, spaghetti, alcohol and devitalized foods, raise merry hell in your gastrointestinal tract, *lactose* is a well-behaved little carbohydrate. Lactose does not ferment, causing gas and after-meal distress, nor does it irritate the stomach membrane as the other artificial carbohydrates are likely to do.

Lactose is one of the few carbohydrates that actually does several beneficial things for your body. It acts as a choline-sparer, that is, it makes a little choline do the work of more; it promotes the building up of riboflavin, pyridoxine and niacin in the intestine; it also promotes your body's absorption of calcium and phosphorus. And, very important, lactose aids the growth of the highly desirable acidophilus bacteria in your intestinal tract—bacteria which help keep it in good working order, preventing the growth of unwanted fungi and bacteria among fermenting food residues.

Lactose is a youth-promoter, too, because it provides a quick, readily usable source of energy for older bodies that need every iota of energy they can muster to counteract a slowing down of the nervous system and the vital organs.

It has long been known that some foods stimulate the sex glands. Among the more commonly recognized of such foods are eggs, oysters and red meats. Their is another that should be added to the list—*milk*.

Mahatma Gandhi, world-famous holy man of India, in later years after taking his vow of continence sought to repress his normal sexual desires. As part of his self-imposed ascetic life, he also limited his diet to fruits and nuts. But after a while he discovered that this extremely limited diet did not provide the strength he needed to carry on his vigorous campaigns of non-resistance among his countrymen (resulting in long imprisonments for himself), so he was obliged to add milk to his daily meals.

Now, while he had been subsisting on nothing except fruits and nuts, the Mahatma reported experiencing no difficulty in maintaining his vow of abstinence from sex. But, almost as soon as he started drinking milk each day, he noticed that his sexual desires became increasingly stronger. The Mahatma's experience with milk and sex has been borne out by many past-forty persons who report strengthened sexual powers after adding liberal amounts of high-protein foods to their everyday diet.

Milk, like other high-protein foods, contains factors of great importance to the human organs of reproduction.

We know that protein, calcium, riboflavin and thiamine exert an important influence on the continued youthfulness of the sex glands in men and women alike. Laboratory research has demonstrated that liberal amounts of these four nutrients in the daily diet can prolong sexual desires. Powdered milk was the food used in the experiment to provide the added qualities of these four nutrition elements.

It was learned that the laboratory animal could be nourished well enough to remain alive and active on a diet of five parts of whole wheat to one part of milk powder. But when the milk powder was increased *from one-fifth to one-third* of the entire mixture, not only was there a definite increase in sexual powers, but in general health and longevity as well.

A British scientist advocated not long ago that all married couples, whatever their ages, should look to their diets if they wished to achieve a congenial marital partnership. The quarrelsome mate is quite likely to be one whose nerves are starved for protein, calcium and the B-vitamins, especially thiamine. The "frigid" wife, or the sexually indifferent husband, is probably one whose sex organs are too undernourished because of improper diet to be capable of their full powers.

This thought-provoking fact is brought before you at this point because it has long been my belief that the lopsided, artificial, woefully devitalized diets of a great majority of American families create the real causes underlying so much unhappy married life. The love and harmony of marriage are severely strained by "on-edge" nerves, and an irregular, indifferent sex life. Many marriages grow old sexually long before the husband or the wife. And the partner to a sexless marriage, whether he or she will admit it openly, has a feeling of lost youth that turns the joy of living to bitterest gall.

So whatever you can do to retain the sexual youthfulness of your marriage is an important step toward guarding your own self against premature aging in mind and body alike.

Certainly I don't want to give the impression that powdered milk is going to cure all the ills of your marriage. But I do want you to consider the logic of safeguarding your marital happiness by making certain that your nervous system and your sexual glands are well fortified by protective foods so you can retain the youthfulness necessary for a prolonged period of normal sex enjoyment.

Is there a real need for dried skim milk? With more than half of the people losing their youth before they are forty, I should say there is.

Chapter 12

HONEY BELONGS ON YOUR TABLE

PLEASE don't get the idea that because I warn so constantly against the evils of white sugar, I am against all sweets in your Eat-and-Grow-Younger diet. I enjoy a sweet as much as you. But I try to confine these sweet sprees to a type of carbohydrate that will make a definite contribution to my daily nutrition—that is, to confections and desserts made with pure honey. These are natural sweets, and not the sickly product of a white sugar refinery.

You probably need no introduction to the goodness of nuts and fresh or dried fruits. And you already know that both unrefined raw sugar and unsulphured syrups are fair sources of minerals. But your sole knowledge of *honey* may consist of the one fact that it is "made by bees."

Perhaps you've never been told that honey is the only *animal carbohydrate* available to us as a sweet; that it is the only *predigested* sugar in nature, being 99 per cent predigested when it reaches your table. Although the *dextrose* or *levulose* (sometimes called "grape sugar" or "blood sugar") in honey is the sweetest of all sugars, it is also the mildest, the easiest to digest and the best source of quick, lasting energy.

Honey is one of the few sweets that possess natural laxative properties. It is also one of the quickest stimulants known. Half an ounce (one tablespoon) of honey in a cup of hot water is one of the fastest-acting restoratives in cases of shock, fainting or after a hemorrhage. Moreover, the use of honey in the diet as a sweetener does not result in the heavy production of body fat that follows the use of 100-per-cent starch, no-vitamin, no-mineral white sugar.

Honey made by the bees from the nectar of flowers has a high vitamin C content. But, to retain its vitamin C content, the honey must not be heated or too highly strained. The darker the honey, the more nutrition it contains, although the flavor of the light-colored honeys is somewhat milder. Not only does honey contain vitamin C, but it also retains this easily destroyed vitamin longer than most fruits and vegetables which lose their vitamin C rather quickly after exposure to air and heat.

Most honeys can also supply your diet with thiamine and riboflavin, (along with other B-vitamins) and a good proportion of food minerals, plus some hormones, and a few amino acids (protein), together with diastase and other enzymes that help digestion. Can the same be said of white sugar? Indeed not! You get nothing but pure starch when you buy white sugar—and your problem is how to cut down on starches, not increase them.

When you adopt honey as your principal Eat-and-Grow-Younger sweetener, you'll be using a sweet that has already won its medals from nutritional science. For honey is universally recognized as a *protective* food. The *Swiss Bee Journal* reports an experiment conducted in that country with three groups of children, all in poor health. The first group was given a normal diet; the second group was given a normal diet plus medication; while the third group was fed the same diet *plus honey*. The honey-fed group of sickly children "outdistanced the other two in every respect: blood count, weight, energy, vivacity and general appearance."

Honey, as a supreme conditioner for strenuous activity, was appreciated in ancient times. The unparalleled athletes of ancient Greece trained for their Olympic games on honey. And today mountain climbers and long-distance swimmers use large amounts of honey in their training diets.

Deep-sea divers, too, have learned that honey gives them the energy needed for their grueling work.

European physicians, profiting by the experience of the ages, prescribe honey freely as a medicine. Yet it's somewhat ironic to note that in this country of constant medical research we accord honey only a minor role in medicine, merely as a base for cough syrups into which are compounded various drugs that may, or may not, relieve the cough—but which certainly do harm the stomach! Entirely concealed from the patient is the fact that the honey alone, without the drugs, mixed with a little lemon juice is an excellent remedy for simple coughs.

Dr. Arnold Lorand, the eminent nutrition expert, has this to say about the use of honey as an ideal food for the heart muscle:

"As the best food for the heart, I recommended honey . . . Honey is easily digested and assimilated; it is the best sweet food, as it does not cause flatulence and can prevent it, to a certain extent promoting the activity of the bowels. It can easily be added to the five meals a day I recommend in cases of arteriosclerosis and weak heart. As it would be unwise to leave such a hard-working organ as the heart without any food over the long hours of the night, I recommend heart patients to take before going to bed a glass of water with honey and lemon juice in it, and also to take it when awakening at night. Before and after muscular exertion honey should be given in a generous dose . . . The use of sugar cannot replace honey. In the same amount, sugar is chemically irritating to the stomach."

Nor is Dr. Lorand the only European physician who recognizes the value of honey as a heart food. Dr. G. N. W. Thomas of Edinburgh had this to say about honey in *The Lancet*, most important British medical journal:

"In heart weaknesses I have found honey to have a marked effect in reviving the heart action and keeping patients alive. I have further evidence of this in a recent case of pneumonia. The patient consumed two pounds of honey during the illness; there was a marked early crisis with no subsequent rise in temperature and an exceptionally good pulse. I suggest that honey should be given for general physical repair and, above all, for heart failure."

There is an easily proved, wholly scientific reason why honey is a wonderful food to build quick energy in run-down bodies, to promptly stimulate fatigued bodies back to normal, and to feed weakened heart muscles:

Honey contains as its prime ingredient the sugar *dextrose* which is readily converted in the body to *glycogen*. Now, glycogen is the only form in which sugar can be stored in the human body (main storage places are the liver, gland cells and muscles) for ready use when energy is needed. Every bite of carbohydrate you eat (flour, bread, cake, spaghetti, rice, white sugar, candy, chocolate) must first be broken down in your intestinal tract to dextrose—a long and intricate process. For it is only as dextrose that these carbohydrate foods can pass through the portal vein into the liver to be converted into body sugar or *glycogen*.

If this seems a little too technical, I'll slow down a bit, since it's important that you understand these bodily chemical processes so you may better appreciate the inestimable value of honey in your Eat-and-Grow-Younger diet.

You have heard the expression "blood sugar level" many times. What it means is that a certain amount of glycogen must be present in your bloodstream at all times; otherwise the efficiency of your body grows less and less. In cases of a severely decreased blood sugar level (insulin shock, brought on by an overdose of the diabetes treatment, is one instance), the brain slows down so completely that the person goes into a deep coma; and death is the result when the level of glycogen in the blood falls too low to maintain life any longer.

In a much milder form, a lowered blood sugar level is what causes you to seek a between-meals snack when you begin feeling brain-and-body tired.

Whenever your blood sugar falls to such a low level that it needs raising almost instantly to counteract severe fatigue and a general slowing down of the heart muscle, would you be wise in eating a food that requires a long, intricate digestive processing before it can be turned into the dextrose that produces the instantly usable glycogen? Or should you choose a food that is already a *99 per cent pre-digested dextrose?* That means *honey.*

When you depend on other carbohydrates for energy (the lactose in milk is the one exception), your heart muscle, your brain cells, your bloodstream must all wait for that urgently needed glycogen until the long, intricate digestive process is finished.

Not so with honey. Almost on the instant, needed amounts of glycogen appear in the bloodstream after this natural sweet is eaten. Those deep-sea divers mentioned above did not restore their severely depleted energy by eating a candy bar, or by coffee and doughnuts. Quick-acting honey was the unfailing energizer they depended on to give them the strength to complete their grueling tasks.

In addition to being an unexcelled energy food, honey is also one of nature's most powerful germ killers. Germs simply cannot survive in honey. A long series of experiments by bacteriologists in this country and in Canada have proved that bacteria introduced into honey always die within a very short time.

The germ that causes typhoid fever, as well as that which results in inflammation of the intestines, died after forty-eight hours when left in pure honey; and the micro-organisms responsible for dysentery were destroyed in ten hours.

Not only is honey itself the purest of foods, it is also a good purifier for your digestive tract.

The Slavic peoples, as well as the Greeks, Italians and Hungarians, consider honey an excellent laxative, using it also as a remedy for coughs, bronchitis, and simple lung disorders. Honey is also an efficient diuretic, that is, it increases the production and discharge of urine. For this reason, honey has been used since ancient times as a dependable remedy for many kidney and bladder disorders.

Persons suffering from the very painful ailment called *pyelitis* (an inflammation of the lower kidney) show speedy improvement when given honey, because this natural medicine increases the amount of urine and exerts a pronounced antiseptic effect on the inflamed area.

My own nutritional studies have convinced me that honey is particularly valuable as a sweetener in the diet of anyone past the age of forty, since it places no burden on the digestion. Honey cannot ferment in the digestive tract (as does white sugar and all the foods made with it), and therefore honey does not set up those ideal conditions for the growth of harmful bacteria as do partially digested high-starch foods. For this one reason alone, no better tonic than honey could be added to the diet of convalescents and persons of advanced years.

Further, I have investigated several cases of stomach and intestinal irritations that did not respond well to any other treatment, but which cleared up when treated with routine use of a tea made from the seeds of the fenugreek herb liberally sweetened with pure honey.

I also have knowledge of many arthritic persons who have obtained a most heartening relief after replacing white sugar in their cooked and uncooked foods with liberal amounts of honey.

As the use of refined white sugar has increased during the past 150 years, replacing the honey which formerly had been the poor man's sweetener (processed sugar was very expensive and only royalty or the wealthy class could afford it), medical statistics kept on recording the steady growth of new, and often fatal, digestive and nervous diseases among the people of the English-speaking world.

Dr. Harvey Wiley, former director of the Bureau of Foods of the U. S. Department of Agriculture, urged that the use of white sugar be abandoned because of its health-destroying effects, and that honey be universally restored as a sweetener. Dr. F. G. Banting, the scientist who discovered insulin as a treatment for diabetes, warned that refined sugar was a "dangerous foodstuff."

Honey is the outstanding natural sweet to use in infant feeding. Tolerated by most babies, it furnishes the baby with a sweet, minerals supplementing those found in milk, a small amount of protein, an antiseptic, and a mild laxative. The minerals found in honey provide the infant with part of the needs of a growing body. They include copper, iron, silicon, manganese, calcium, chlorine, sodium, potassium, sulphur, phosphorus, and magnesium.

Two or more teaspoonfuls of honey with each meal will insure adequate honey nutrients for your body needs. The honeybee gives you many valid nutritional reasons for including the product of his chemistry in your diet.

Honey is rich in the B vitamins. H. A. Schuette of the University of Wisconsin's Department of Chemistry, one of the outstanding investigators of vitamins in honey, described his determination of the B vitamins in honey in the *Journal of Nutrition*. Results of all the honeys examined showed the following presence of B-complex vitamins per 100 grams:

Riboflavin—7 to 60 micrograms

Pantothenic acid—9 to 110 micrograms

Niacin—72 to 590 micrograms

Thiamine—1.4 to 12 micrograms

Pyridoxine—up to 27.7 micrograms

Traces of biotin and folic acid were also found in some of the honeys tested. The researchers discovered that the vitamin content of pollen is much higher than that of honey. For this reason, clarifying honey *reduces* the vitamin content by as much as 50 per cent of the original values.

Varying also with the kind of honey, and the locality from which it comes, is the vitamin C content: Up to 311.2 milligrams per 100 grams have been found, greatly exceeding the vitamin C content of an orange weighing 100 grams.

In further experiments, Dr. Schuette found that honey contains 14 to 72 milligrams per kilogram of copper; 2.4 to 17.5 of iron; .29 to 1.4 of silicon; up to 58 of phosphorus; 5 to 226 of calcium; 7 to 126 magnesium. Darker honeys, generally, had a higher mineral content than light.

With its enzymes, honey can aid digestion; yet honey itself requires no process of digestion before it can be utilized by the body. Honey has been found to stimulate the flow of various salivary and digestive secretions, as well as to aid in the building of certain tissues.

Honey has been known to aid in the functioning of the ductless glands, chiefly the thyroid, and experiments are now under way to determine the amount and type of hormones it contains. The effect of the dark, *unstrained* honeys on arthritics has led some experimenters to believe it may contain some hormone other than an infinitesimally small amount of bee venom.

Beekeeper Mrs. B of Michigan said her arthritic pains disappeared when she helped her husband extract honey. The pains reappeared as soon as she was not working in the apiary.

A German physician, Dr. Heerman, advances the theory that the internal use of honey is just as effective in treating arthritis and kindred ailments as the bee sting. It may be that this mysterious sting substance, which so far has defied chemical analysis, supplies the effect for treatment of arthritis, rheumatism, and gout.

I have devoted an entire chapter to acquainting you with honey because I believe that you would be well-advised to adopt pure, unstrained honey as your most important sweet food.

Professor McCollum of Johns Hopkins University includes honey *among our best protective foods*. And Elie Metchnikoff, the famous Russian scientist, attributes the unusually *long life* of Bulgarian peasants to their milk-and-honey diet.

Dr. Rubner of the University of Berlin, an eminent nutritional physiologist, has corroborated H. A. Schuette's findings that *honey contains an abundance of the important B-vitamins.*

But, best of all—like all the other youth-protecting foods in my Eat-and-Grow-Younger diet—honey *tastes good.* It makes mealtime and snacktime a pleasure, not an endurance contest.

Chapter 13

THE SURE WAY TO GOOD LOOKS AND CHARM

DURING my stay in Buenos Aires, I was a guest at a formal dinner party in one of the old Argentine mansions. My host was the elder brother of my *estanciero* friend who raised thoroughbred horses, and on whose *estancia* I had met those marvelous old Gauchos saluted in an earlier chapter.

The guests were a cosmopolitan group made up of an English couple, several Argentineans, a Brazilian scientist and his wife, a Uruguayan diplomat, a visiting Italian general and a French count and countess.

The evening hadn't progressed very far when I noticed the French countess, an extremely attractive woman, speaking earnestly with our host who singled me out with his glance, then nodded, apparently in answer to some question of hers concerning me. Immediately the countess came over to me.

"Monsieur Kordel," she said, "how old would you think me?"

I was taken aback by this abrupt question. It's not good policy to play at age-guessing games with the ladies, no matter how charming and youthful they may be. A guess of a year or two too many, and one really has blundered!

I looked closely at her clear, fresh skin, her sparkling gray eyes, and her lustrous dark brown hair. She could have been anywhere between thirty and a youthful forty. Her figure was well-rounded without being lumpy, and her carriage was remarkably graceful. So I waded in with my best guess.

"Thirty-three, perhaps. And surely not more than thirty-five."

She gave me a searching look. "Yes, I believe you are being honest. Well, monsieur, last month I celebrated—yes, that is the right word, *celebrated*—my fifty-third birthday! I have a son as old as you guessed me!"

She called her husband, who extracted from his wallet a small, worn photograph and passed it to me. It was a picture of a woman, quite evidently a relative of the countess, for the features showed a marked resemblance to hers. Yet this was a much older woman.

"That, Monsieur Kordel," she said, "was my face five years ago, before we left France."

"It's hard to believe," I said. "This woman looks a good fifty-five, if not more."

"And so I did!" she agreed.

Quite apparently there was an exciting story behind the incredible rejuvenation of a woman who had looked every one of her middle-aged years into an attractive creature who could have passed for her own much younger sister.

I glanced closely at her face. It bore none of the telltale traces ordinarily left by a face-lifting operation. Still, everyone knows how clever are the plastic surgeons who practice their art in Paris. Yet, even so, a mechanical rejuvenation of the facial muscles cannot possible restore sparkle to dull eyes, or sheen to lifeless hair.

"I was about to guess plastic surgery," I admitted frankly. "But there most certainly is more to your secret than a face-lifting operation."

Her laugh was delightful, the laugh of a truly happy woman. The count joined in her laughter, then addressed me.

"The 'secret,' monsieur," he said, "is one you also share. My wife has been a zealous follower of your teachings on nutrition since arriving in Buenos Aires in 1946. An American friend loaned her a copy of your book. And from that day it has become the book of rules for our kitchen. No dish on the menu unless Heloise is certain it has so many grams of protein, such-and-such minerals, so many vitamins."

The countess broke in smiling. "I'm not quite the tyrant you say! But sincerely, Monsieur Kordel, when I read your book it came like a great revelation to me. Always in France we have eaten for the sheer pleasure of it, never thinking what harm all those rich foods did to our appearance. Or whether we were fully nourished. But now, with the so plentiful meat of this country and its delicious cheeses, fruits and vegetables, I have found a new *plainer* way of eating . . . And I have found the youth I lost many years ago in France."

She turned toward her husband. "You, too, Georges, how much younger you look than when we left France. Only you, vain one, were too wise to have a photograph made then!"

If only I could bring this *young* middle-aged woman as "Exhibit A" into the beauty salons where women spend fortunes each year to be massaged, creamed and dyed back to a semblance of their former youthful attractiveness—*and all the while they are eating or dieting (even smoking to stifle their normal appetite) themselves into a prematurely aged ap-*

pearance that even the most expensive beauty treatments can never conceal.

Firm muscles, smooth complexions, bright eyes and thick hair are the health-right of every man and woman—not of these alone who can afford to cater to expensive beauty salons, and so-called "muscle-developing" and "hair-restoring" establishments.

All these outward attributes of a prolonged youth can be yours, if you start to work *inwardly* on attaining them. Muscle "developers," beauty creams, wrinkle eradicators and hair tonics are, at best, only stop-gap measures; they cannot *feed* the muscles, the skin, the hair.

You must *reverse* the abnormal chemical reactions in your body that produce flabby muscles, sallow and unduly wrinkled skins, dull eyes and grayed, thinning hair. But first you must understand why these unwelcome signs of a premature age begin to show up decades too soon in most persons. That is what I shall explain to you in the next few chapters, plus outlining for you the recommended diet regimen that can help you regain the vital attractiveness associated with youth.

The same diet regimen, by the way, that was followed to the letter by a well-known author who happens to have been a health student of mine for several years.

This author, whose detective stories have entertained thousands of persons on two continents with their clever, resourceful heroes and courageous heroines, found himself becoming old-looking much too soon for his peace of mind. As he phrases his dilemma: "I could save my fiction offspring from horrible deaths a dozen times a chapter, yet I wasn't able to prevent the steadily approaching death of my own youth. That set me to thinking." And after he had thought seriously about his problem, he came to the conclusion that he didn't know enough about his own body to solve the mystery of his vanishing youth. Whereupon he sought more knowledge, and became a regular attendant at my lectures whenever I appeared in his city. He says that all my previous books and pamphlets on nutrition have become his "textbooks" on youth preservation.

"Not only do I look and feel a whole lot younger," he told me, "but I'm doing better writing these days with a lot less drain on my nervous energy. In the old days I was able to keep myself going at the typewriter only by drinking cups and cups of black coffee, and smoking one cigarette after another. Then, after the manuscript was finished and the letdown came, I was like a caged beast. My nerves went to pieces with a bang, and I wouldn't be any good for months."

He is now feeling and *looking* younger than he ever thought possible for his fifty-eight years.

The average person of middle age—and many younger people—exists on a diet woefully deficient on almost every nutritional count (proteins, minerals, vitamins), unless a conscious effort is made for *planned diet*. Small wonder, then, that good looks and charm are so rare past forty. And small wonder that this early loss of vitality and youthful appearance is particularly true of men, since they need even greater amounts of the B-vitamins (paramount factors in helping your youth stay on the job) than women.

Yet how many men at this critical period in life make a conscious effort to guard against losing the sensations and appearances of youth in the only sure way—through a planned diet? Too few, I'm afraid. All too often the convert to a planned diet is the woman of the family, and her efforts to make friend husband realize the dietary facts behind his loss of energy and youthful appearance meet with indifference, if not open derision.

And yet men are as vain of their good looks and youthful attractions as are women. They may not admit that their appearance matters as much to their happiness as it does to a woman. But I, as one of the "stronger sex," will admit it for them. We men do care—and how!—when the signs of age begin to sreak up on us. Otherwise, why all the hue and cry when a "sure cure" for baldness appears periodically in the headlines; or how else account for the perennial prosperity of the "health establishments" where paunchy business and professional men attempt to defeat a premature old age by enduring strenuous exercises, massages and steam baths that actually harm their undernourished hearts?

In the preceding chapters I have dwelt at length on the paramount need in every diet for plenty of protein—meat, fish, fowl, eggs, cheese, low-fat milk and seed cereals. But I have saved until now the full story of the youth-bestowing B-vitamins because they enter so frequently into any mention of "diet and good looks."

All the youth-preserving members of the B-complex family are found in varying degrees in meats, fish, fowl, eggs, low-fat milk, cheese, seed cereals (like millet, sunflower seeds and sesame seeds), green vegetables, legumes, whole grains, berries, melons and fresh fruits. Wheat germ (the *raw* product found mostly in health food stores, and not the sugared variety found on grocery shelves) is another good source of the B-vitamins.

The full story on millet and dry skim milk is told in

Chapters 10 and 11. But a generous mention of these two foods belongs in any advice on "diet and good looks," because both are unusually rich sources of *riboflavin*, the B-vitamin so everlastingly concerned with the health of your eyes, your skin, your hair. Any noticeable change for the worse in the appearance or health of these features should be an immediate warning that there's not enough riboflavin in the diet.

Here's what usually happens when your body is skimped on riboflavin: Your elbows may become red and wrinkled; the skin over your entire body may coarsen, with a quick tendency toward rashes and other forms of skin disorders. Your hair may grow dull and fall out readily. Unsightly fingernails—split, grooved or fissured—often disappear after the body receives enough riboflavin. If you suddenly develop an abnormally oily complexion, more than likely it's because you need more riboflavin in your diet. Because riboflavin acts on the muscles and nerves of the eyes, a serious lack of this B-vitamin will bring on visual disorders, not the least of which is cataract.

I cannot stress too emphatically the importance of abundant riboflavin in the diet of every person past the age of forty. Symptoms of riboflavin deficiencies are so widespread among persons in this age group that obtaining enough of this B-vitamin is one of the major nutritional problems from middle age onward.

From recent work being done in the nutritional laboratories, I believe that regular use in the diet of millet as well as daily use of powdered skim milk can easily solve the problem of too-little-riboflavin in an *economical* and *tasty* way.

Keeping in mind all the listed food sources of the important B-vitamins, let's go on in the following chapters to discover how this hard-working vitamin family affects your beauty and attractiveness at any age, but especially after you've blown out the candles on your fortieth birthday cake.

Chapter 14

DO YOUR EYES LOOK YOUNG?

DULL, strained, bloodshot, heavily pouched eyes can give you that "lost youth" look quicker than any other feature. Beauty advisers continually admonish their readers to avoid the frowning, strained expressions caused by tired, dull, undernourished eyes.

No optician has yet invented a pair of eyeglasses that will restore beauty and sparkle to dull, undernourished eyes. You may bolster up your dimming vision with these mechanical aids, but eyeglasses certainly can't do anything to bolster your good looks and charm. I don't mean by this that you should cast aside your glasses. But I do say that you shouldn't perch a pair of glasses in front of your eyes, and then expect these purely external aids to bring your eyes back to the bright, sparkling beauty that only good health can give them.

Any unhealthy condition (and premature aging is most assuredly an unhealthy condition) of the body is quickly reflected both *in* the eyes, and *under* them. Nothing detracts more from a person's appearance of youth than darkly circled eyes.

Dark, puffy pouches are caused by the condition of the skin underneath the eye socket. In this area the skin differs from that in other parts of the body. Pinch the skin on your arm, your thigh, your cheek, and you'll discover that a layer of fatty padding lies directly below the surface. But the skin covering the lower half of the eye cavity is much thinner and lacks this basic under layer of fat.

The difference in skin texture has been arranged by nature to guarantee protection for the eyes, since the skin of the eyelids and that under the eyes themselves must be extremely flexible to permit quick, effortless blinking. Obviously, if the skin around the eyes were as thick and as bulky as that in other parts of the body it would be impossible to wink quickly enough to protect the eyes when foreign substances threaten.

And because the skin under the eyes is so thin the condition of the blood flowing in this semi-transparent area may readily be detected. Healthy blood is naturally red, whereas blood darkened by impurities, lack of sleep or improper food immediately discolors the skin over the lower eye socket. So if you allow yourself to become—and remain—anemic because of an iron-deficient diet, you can expect the bluish type of low-hemoglobin blood that makes ugly dark circles under the eyes (not to mention the other uncomfortable, youth-destroying effects of anemia).

The high-starch foods (white breads, macaroni, spaghetti, noodles, white rice, pastries, cakes, heavy puddings, candies, soft drinks, alcohol) have a tendency to increase the amount of carbon dioxide in the blood, causing it to lose its rich, red color. This explains why a diet top-heavy with these artificial, high-starch foods and beverages can hasten the appearance of those unsightly, aging dark circles under the eyes.

On the other hand, fruits, particularly citrus fruits, fresh green and yellow vegetables, and the iron-rich foods that make good red blood (see Chapter 18) are the foods that will help clear up dark circles under the eyes, and guard against their reappearance. Not only will these nourishing foods cause the dark circles to fade, but your eyes themselves will gain an added sparkle from the richer blood built up by a planned diet.

The full story of *vitamin A and healthy eyes* was too well publicized during World War II with the Government's "carrots for aviators" program to need repeating here at length. Just a reminder that vitamin A not only corrects night blindness, but also protects against an ailment that causes a dry, thickened condition of the eyelid itself, leaving the eyeball lusterless and diseased. And if the foods you eat do not provide enough vitamin A to keep the tear ducts healthy, the eyes cannot secrete enough of the moisture that lubricates the eyeball and helps impart to it that glistening, sparkling look so necessary for attractive young-looking eyes.

At the University of Georgia, a study was made of 47 persons known to be suffering from a lack of riboflavin in their diets. All 47 of these riboflavin-deficient persons complained of trouble with their eyes—sensitivity to light, dim vision, an eyestrain which glasses did not remedy, burning sensations in the eyeball, extreme visual fatigue, a feeling of roughness like sand under the eyelids, watering, and bloodshot eyeballs.

But a marked improvement was noted in the eyes of all 47 patients after *5 to 15 milligrams of riboflavin* were added to their diets each day. In many cases, the sensitivity to light disappeared in only twenty-four hours. And the burning, itching and feeling of roughness under the lids cleared up within two days.

Take a look at your eyes in the mirror. If they are even slightly bloodshot, you can be pretty certain they need more riboflavin. Under normal conditions the thin covering over the entire eye contains no blood vessels. Nature devised a clever way of bringing oxygen to the outer eye without the need for a disfiguring network of blood vessels—the riboflavin in the blood back of the eye combines with oxygen in the air to supply the part of your eyeball that is visible.

But what happens to this ingenious oxygen-supplying system if there isn't enough riboflavin in the blood back of the eyes? Then nature sets up a second-best system by creating small blood vessels to bring oxygen directly to the outer eye tissues.

It's when a lack of riboflavin makes nature resort to this makeshift oxygen-carrying measure that your eyes are said to be *bloodshot,* as indeed they are—shot through with tiny, newly created blood vessels. And who can look young and attractive, no matter how few or how many their birthdays, when the eyes suffer this disfigurement?

Although "spots before the eyes" in the earlier years rarely have any particular significance other than that of nervousness, from the middle years onward they should be heeded as a warning that all may not be well with the eye.

"Cataract" is a word dreaded more and more as the years accumulate. And rightly so, for this is a serious disease of the eye that clouds the tiny lens inside the eye.

When only skimpy amounts of riboflavin are supplied to your eyes, you may be laying the foundation for cataracts—and when this lack of riboflavin is coupled with an inadequacy of the high-protein foods needed to provide ample quantities of certain amino acids, then ideal conditions are set up for the ocular lens to become clouded.

Since a planned diet can *avoid* the danger of cataract blindness, why take chances? The common type of so-called "senile" cataract that is brought on when the eye starves for riboflavin and high proteins is just as damaging to your eyesight—and to your appearance—as the cataract caused by an eye injury.

Almost every disturbance in the chemistry of your body may first make itself evident in your eyes. This is why many competent diagnosticians begin their hunt for symptoms with a thorough examination of the eye itself. Eyes that tire easily or become painful and bleary may mean that the blood sugar level is too high, that the blood formation is below normal, or that the liver is sluggish. These and other ailments can be noted first in the eyes, the body's "radar" for disease-finding.

This explains why I deplore the careless practice of considering any change in vision as a matter solely within the province of the eyeglass fitter.

No pair of lenses, no matter how skillfully prescribed or ground, can arrest the progress of an eye disease; they cannot provide nourishment for a starving eye; nor can eyeglasses clear up the bowel and gall bladder disorders that react directly upon the eyes, to say nothing of that master sight-dimmer, diabetes.

Toxic materials filtering into the bloodstream from starch-clogged intestines, or backing up from a disordered gall bladder and liver, make it difficult for the eyes to focus properly since they are being poisoned by the waste-laden blood which normally is supposed to nourish and cleanse them of their own impurities.

You didn't know there was any connection between your eyes and your bowels? Well, there certainly is!

A doctor whom I met some years ago had been a victim of chronic constipation for years. By the time he reached his sixtieth year, his eyes finally gave up the struggle, and refused to focus, even behind the strongest lenses he could buy.

Knowing the antagonism that many of the medical profession show toward nutrition scientists, I hesitated to suggest what I was sure would relieve his failing vision. But I decided to take a chance anyhow.

Surprisingly enough, he listened readily to my suggestions, no doubt scared by the thought of total blindness into taking advice from a "non-medical" man.

Here is what I told him: "Do away with all those high-starch foods I know you eat, for I've sat at the table and watched you stuffing them down. Confine your meals to high protein foods like meat, fish, poultry, eggs, cheese, low-fat milk, and seed cereals. Round out this diet with whole grains, fresh and cooked fruits, and leafy, low-carbohydrate vegetables. Don't cheat! Then let me hear in about six months how you're getting along."

Seven months later, to the day, I received this letter from him: "You didn't think I'd do it, but I did! My bowels and I have reached an amicable working agreement. I don't choke them up with starchy foods any more, so they let my eyes alone. Life, it's wonderful—when your bowels and your eyes let you enjoy it!"

Chapter 15

DON'T INVITE "OLD" HAIR AND SKIN

IT'S a toss up which does more to help you retain the appearance of youth—a head of thick, lustrous hair or a smooth skin, glowing with health.

Let's first diagnose what's wrong when your hair begins to "show its age."

The absence from your diet of no one single nutrient is wholly responsible when your hair becomes dry, discolored, lusterless, and begins to grow thinner, coming out "by the handfuls." Nutritional science has proved that this unhealthy state happens whenever several different food elements are lacking in your diet.

Because each single hair is made of *protein*, your hair needs the sulphur-supplying amino acids found in egg yolk. (This also holds good for healthy fingernails.) When you don't eat enough of these particular amino acids, your hair becomes lusterless and lacks sheen. It's a well-known trick among horse fanciers to feed a show horse on eggs so his coat will acquire that beautiful sheen so greatly admired in a prize animal. And egg shampoos have long been a popular beauty treatment for human hair.

The only fault I can find with this beauty treatment is that the egg is wasted on the outside—*eat* your eggs for beautiful hair with a sheen!

This brings protein into our growing list of nutrients that feed your hair. But what about vitamins?

Science has discovered that there is a mysterious pact between these three—proteins, minerals and vitamins. A sort of "closed shop" agreement whereby neither of the group will perform to its greatest or most efficient capacity unless the other two are there in full force.

The first vitamin in this "hair pact" is vitamin A—the same fellow that feeds your eyes and helps keep them in good seeing order. If your diet is not providing enough vitamin A, then you may expect dry, dead-looking hair, with a scalp well powdered with dandruff. And if you permit this vitamin deficiency to become more severe, your hair will grow coarse and ugly, then begin falling out.

Next are these B-vitamins—*pantothenic acid, para-amino-benzoic acid* and *inositol*.

Pantothenic acid became known several years ago as "the gray hair vitamin." A fad of taking this isolated vitamin in concentrated doses swept over the country. Beauty parlors became dispensaries of pantothenic acid capsules, while barbers began urging their male customers to buy them. As a result, hundreds of persons began religiously taking their "gray hair vitamin." Some noticed what they reported as a slight improvement in the coloration of their hair, but the great majority were frank to admit that it "didn't do much good." Why?

Because experience has now taught us that no single food element can work its nutritional wonders toward keeping us healthy and young-looking when isolated from its cohorts.

That is, when separated from the other members of its own family, as well as from certain other vital food elements.

In the case of the "gray hair vitamin" fad, pantothenic acid was sent out to do its job without para-aminobenzoic and inositol, all three of them being members of the same B-complex family where nature placed them, each to complement and round out the work of the others.

That is why pure pantothenic acid capsules failed in a great majority of cases to restore color to gray hair—because one vitamin was expected to handle the task normally performed by *three B-vitamins,* aided by protein and certain minerals, all working as a team.

I've saved until last the story of *inositol and baldness* as a sort of encouragement "dividend" for you men.

Dr. Wooley of Rockefeller Institute has linked a deficiency of inositol directly to baldness. In an extensive experiment he fed laboratory animals a diet that was adequate in every respect, *except* it didn't contain any inositol whatsoever. Before long, the hair on these animals began falling out until large patches on their bodies became completely bald. But when he started feeding them either concentrated inositol or the natural vitamin as found in foods rich in the B-vitamins, the bald patches were covered with a complete new growth of hair in only eighteen days.

Now, I'm not promising that you'll grow a new thatch in eighteen days if you add inositol to your diet. Throughout this book, as in all my books, I avoid extravagant claims. But I can tell you that many persons who have taken the precaution to add to their planned diets generous amounts of the delicious foods rich in all the B-vitamins have been delighted to notice a distinct growth of new hair.

The question is often asked why men become bald more readily than women.

A variety of stock phrases is always on hand to answer this perfectly logical question—hereditary tendencies, tight hats, too frequent shampooing, greater sexual activity and so forth. Yet seldom does anyone give the one provable answer: *Men need even greater quantities of the important B-vitamins than do women, hence their more serious lack of these food elements reacts on their scalps.*

In our enlightened era of milling the youth-preserving B-vitamins out of our grains and our sugar cane, it is the men who suffer the more acute deficiencies of inositol. So why don't you men concentrate on keeping your hair through feeding it, rather than dousing it with costly, worthless, sweet-smelling hair tonics?

The mineral *chlorine,* when only partially lacking from the diet of laboratory animals, will cause their hair to fall out. This also happens if the trace mineral *zinc* is not amply supplied to these experimental animals: their hair does not develop normally, and is quickly lost. The same is true of *silicon.* Another mineral involved in keeping your hair healthy and "in your scalp" is *iodine.* As I explained in Chapter 8, when not enough iodine is provided the thyroid gland to produce its hormone, one of the unpleasant symptoms is brittle, lifeless hair that falls out too readily and is not amply replaced, resulting in a progressive tendency toward a bare scalp.

Here's a quick resumé of the food elements you should think of as nourishing your hair: *high-grade protein;* vitamin A; the B-vitamins—*pantothenic acid, para-aminobenzoic acid* and *inositol;* and the minerals *iodine, chlorine, silicon* and *zinc.*

Your *skin,* the same as your hair, is made of protein. In fact, it's possible to produce ulcers of the skin merely by keeping the diet extremely low in protein. Yet these skin ulcers can be healed quickly enough when abundant quantities of high-protein foods are restored to the meals.

Similarly, a reducing diet (or any other diet, for that matter) which excludes fats is bound to result in a dry, wrinkled skin. Safflower, sesame and sunflower seed oils contain certain valuable *unsaturated* fatty acids.

A dry, scaly condition of the skin is likely to develop when an *insufficient* amount of these valuable *unsaturated* fatty acids are eaten. These skin-conditioning fatty acids are generously available in the oils mentioned. Or, if you prefer obtaining your daily supply of them by eating the hulled sunflower seeds, that is equally effective. These seeds will also supply two other skin foods—*vitamin A* and *calcium.*

Anyone who has ever traveled in Mediterranean countries where sesame oil "flows like water" has noticed the beautiful smooth skin so prevalent among the women of those countries.

This was also my outstanding impression of the women, both young and old, whom I saw in the South American countries where the Latin use of cooking oils (mainly sunflower seed) is widespread.

I might mention here that sesame oil makes a wonderful skin softener when used instead of the costly, highly perfumed face creams and lotions whose alcoholic content (in the perfumes) tends to dry your skin that much more. The historically famous women of the ancient Mediterranean world learned many centuries ago that sesame oil—used internally, as well as externally—was their best skin beautifier.

Try keeping a small, wide-mouthed jar of pure sesame oil in the bathroom cabinet, and lubricate your skin *lightly* with this natural softener at least once a day. You'll be amazed to notice how the oil soaks into the skin so thoroughly there's no need to wipe off the surplus with a cleansing tissue, thus leaving a fresh dewy softness like that of a true youthful complexion.

While on the subject of external skin beautifiers for the ladies, here is an excellent cosmetic treatment that was standard among the lovely ladies of the ancient world. Mix about two tablespoons of millet meal with a like amount of honey, add about two teaspoons of sesame oil and combine into a smooth paste. After tying the hair well in a cloth or soft towel, apply this paste liberally over the face and neck, keeping well away from the eyes to avoid smarting (not that the mixture is in any way harmful to the eyes). Allow to remain on for at least half an hour, longer if possible. Then wipe off and dash cold water over the skin.

But please don't concentrate on this external aid, and neglect feeding your skin from the *inside*. This excellent beauty mask is nothing more than an adjunct to your beauty diet, to counteract the effects of harsh cosmetics, too much sun, smoky atmospheres, dusty climates, or drying soaps and hard waters. (Remember, also, that a little honey and sesame oil, to which a few drops of rose water are added, can be a wonderful treatment for the roughened skin on your hands, arms and elbows.)

And now to get back to the effects of diet on your skin. If your body, as a whole, is not properly nourished, the skin is usually one of the first organs to show signs of a nutritional deficiency. I know of no quicker way to bring on skin disfigurements of various kinds and seriousness than by loading the diet with a lot of artificial, high-starch foods, and neglecting the proteins, fresh vegetables and fruits.

When the diet does not contain enough *vitamin A,* one of the early symptoms is a pimply eruption which resembles acne. Milder forms have the rough, unsightly appearance of "goose flesh."

Pellagra, the deficiency disease caused by a serious lack of the B-vitamins, *niacin* in particular, is characterized by severe skin troubles, that begin on the hands and feet and resemble a bad sunburn, with blisters and cracked skin.

Biotin, one of the B-vitamins, when seriously lacking in the diet, results in a dry, peeling skin, also causing it to take on a grayish pallor. A word of caution is needed here. Even though you may think your diet contains ample B-complex, if you eat *raw egg white* in meringues, eggnogs, or in other ways, the *avidin* in the uncooked egg white will combine with biotin and prevent this B-vitamin from reaching your bloodstream. Therefore, a biotin deficiency may occur, despite an abundance of B-complex in the diet, if *uncooked* egg white is also included.

When the minerals *iodine* and *iron* are not regularly and adequately supplied to your body, the skin suffers. Too little iodine, of course, slows down production of the thyroid hormone, and one result of this hormone deficiency is an ugly, dry, rough skin. Iron, the mineral so urgently needed by the blood to prevent anemia, gives the skin a smooth, healthy glow which is a reflection of the rich blood flowing through it.

No doubt you're waiting for me to tell you that such-and-such foods will "erase" the wrinkles from your face. That I cannot do and still tell the truth. But I can tell you that a skin which is not allowed to become dry and roughened, either because of external abuse or internal starvation, is far less likely to develop and retain deep wrinkles than a poorly nourished skin.

And I can assure you that wrinkles, in themselves, are not always disfiguring. I'm thinking of those merry laugh and smile wrinkles which give character to a face. Did anyone ever see human warmth or merriment in the wax-smooth, wrinkle-free, expressionless face of a doll? Wrinkles are not seriously detrimental in a face and body that are kept youthful through planned diet.

Far more aging than wrinkles are dull eyes, sallow and jaundiced skin, a weary stoop and creaking gait.

And *wrinkles in the disposition* are more telltale of age than wrinkles in the face.

So if you'll concentrate on restoring smoothness and a healthy color to your skin in the ways I've recommended above, I can assure you that there will be nothing withered about either your skin or your spirit.

Chapter 16

YOUR BONES AND MUSCLES CAN BE TATTLETALES

A FEW years ago while in New York on a lecture tour, I attended a stage performance of a celebrated matinée idol— an actor whose masculine charms have had the ladies sighing and yearning for more years than said idol would publicly admit.

In this particular play, he was portraying the role of an intrepid young explorer. As the curtain went up, he was seated on a log in front of a campfire. The stage lighting cast a flattering glow on his smooth young face, and he ran his hand carelessly over what I suspected was a meticulously marcelled toupee.

"He certainly holds his age well," was my first thought, "even discounting all the make-up tricks."

But just then, at an offstage cue, this apparently well-preserved actor was supposed to leap up from the log and rush to greet an oncoming actor. Yet the best our young-looking matinée idol could manage was a creaky elevation of his stiff body to an upright position. Instantly all illusion of youth was shattered. No toupee or make-up could hide the age in this actor's bones and muscles!

No firmly established law of nature decrees that a man or woman must go creaking and shuffling through the remainder of his or her days after passing a certain age.

Barring serious injury (and even then correct diet can help speed a normal recovery), there's no reason why you should not walk with as firm a step, or arise from a chair with as much grace at seventy as you did at thirty. But you cannot abuse—and by this I mean *starve*—your bones and muscles, and still expect them to provide you with a firm foundation for continuing to look and feel young.

What are the food elements essential to healthy bones?

Most commonly recognized nutrients are *calcium* and *phosphorus*, since we know that our bones are composed mainly of these two minerals. Because you, as an average person, will lose from your body nearly an ounce of these precious minerals every day, constant replacement through the diet is vitally necessary to continued good health and strong bones.

Powdered skim milk, and the various kinds of cheese, particularly cottage cheese, are reliable sources of food calcium, as is sunflower seed meal. Lean meat and eggs are other good sources of calcium as well as protein. Phosphorus, the other "bone mineral," is likewise found in milk, cheese, eggs and lean meat, fish and poultry.

But all the calcium-rich foods and the balanced mineral concentrate you take are not going to do your bones—or the other calcium-craving organs in your body—much good if that calcium cannot reach the bloodstream to be distributed where needed. Two chemical processes in your body may interfere with proper use of food calcium.

As mentioned in earlier chapters, the digestive acids in a normal stomach are composed mainly of hydrochloric acid. It takes the action of *strong* hydrochloric acid to dissolve calcium from foods that reach the stomach so this mineral may be assimilated through the intestinal walls into the bloodstream.

This is also true of other important food minerals such as phosphorus, magnesium and iron. But if the stomach acids are too weak to dissolve the mineral and keep it in solution until it can pass through the intestinal walls into the blood, then the calcium (other minerals, too) moves on through the body, undigested.

Therefore, even though your diet may contain plenty of calcium, none of it will reach your bones (or your heart, muscles, glands and nerves) unless your stomach acids are strong enough to dissolve the mineral and keep it in solution.

There are two ways in which to increase the concentrated acidity of your digestive juices: First, by having your stomach acids tested by a reliable physician, who may then prescribe so many drops of dilute hydrochloric acid to be taken in water with every meal; and second, by adding liberal quantities of vitamin B-complex to your diet, since this group of B-vitamins greatly influences the flow and acidity of your stomach juices.

No mention of calcium and phosphorus for the bones is complete without including *vitamin D,* the "sunshine vitamin." We know that vitamin D, in some mysterious way, controls the retention, absorption and distribution of these minerals in the bones. That is one reason why the serious lack of vitamin D in children will cause rickets, a disease characterized by bowed leg bones, knocked knees, malformed skulls and deformed pelvic bones. And, in adults, a serious lack of vitamin D will hasten the appearance of "brittle" bones.

If you live in a climate where it's possible to be outdoors in the sunshine throughout most of the year, then you need not worry about getting enough vitamin D, since this element is created by the direct action of sunshine on certain oils in your skin.

But if you reside, as most people do, in climates where heavy clothing and indoor living are necessary during six months or so of the year, then your diet should be supplemented during those indoor months by taking a scientifically compounded multiple-vitamin tablet—and by eating a handful of hulled sunflower seeds every day.

Another vitamin that's importantly concerned with keeping your bones young and healthy is *vitamin C*.

Although you may think that your bones remain a constant, unchanged factor in your body structure, this is not true. Your bones continually change, depending upon the quantity of vitamin C you eat from day to day.

During the winter when fresh fruits and vegetables are not abundantly eaten, too little vitamin C is provided your bones, that is, unless you make a special effort to use plenty of citrus fruits, and to supplement the diet with concentrated vitamin C.

This is essential, because without sufficient vitamin C, your bones can be so affected that a fall or a twist which would not result in injury during the summer or late fall, could produce a serious fracture during a long winter when the body's intake of vitamin C was allowed to fall to an abnormally low level.

From this you can appreciate why you should make a conscious effort to keep your diet adequately supplied with vitamin C at all times. Freshly grown and picked vegetables, fruits and melons will supply you with all the vitamin C you need during their season. But if you must depend on market vegetables and fruits, or upon the cooked fruits served in restaurants, then be sure to double the quantity of citrus fruits (eaten *whole*) ordinarily used, and to obtain supplemental amounts through the use of a reliable vitamin concentrate.

Even a partial lack of this important vitamin in the diets of older persons often results in slow, imperfect healing of bone injuries. *At any age, diet plays a major part in the knitting of fractured bones.*

These are the foods which should be abundantly supplied to anyone convalescing from a bone injury of any kind: whole citrus fruits, fresh fruits, berries, melons, green vegetables, pure honey—and, of course, meats, fish, poultry, cheese, milk, eggs and seed cereals for their bone-restoring calcium and phosphorus.

Nor are the vitamins and minerals the only nutrients concerned with keeping your bones young and healing them quickly and properly, if injured. Protein, too, is involved in the bone drama. Large amounts of bone protein are released from the least important muscles whenever a bone fracture occurs so the healing process may take place.

Still another substance that helps control the youthfulness and sturdiness of your bones is *sex hormones*. Maintenance of a healthy skeletal frame for your growing-younger body also depends on how adequate a supply of sex hormones your glands can secrete. (Look to your glands!)

Dr. W. O. Thompson of Chicago reported to the American College of Physicians that supplemental doses of *testosterone* (the male sex hormone) had aided greatly in healing broken bones in elderly men. Dr. Thompson also reported that a marked improvement had been noted in elderly women with broken bones after they had been given estrogen, the female sex hormone.

Laboratory experiments have shown that testosterone helps rebuild muscle and bone substance in *both sexes*. And when this skeletal and muscular balance is maintained throughout the later years, there is less likelihood of developing arthritis, or the physical weakness and disablement resulting from stiffened joints and flabby muscles.

Flabby muscles, whether in the chin or in the legs, are age markers that can destroy all appearance of youthfulness. If the muscles of our aging matinée idol, for example, had retained *tone*, they would have pulled him erect as quickly and as gracefully as the muscles of a twenty-year-old.

Muscle tissues consist almost entirely of protein.

If your body is nourished with a diet built principally around high-protein foods, your muscles have a chance to remain youthfully efficient. If not, then you may expect your muscles to lack *tone*—to become soft and flabby. A body whose muscular system has begun to break down is the body with rounded shoulders, protruding abdomen, drooping head, flabby skin and uncertain gait—all of which detract heavily from your charm and youthful appearance.

Calcium also affects the health and efficiency of your muscles. Irritable muscle tissue is the direct result of too little calcium in the bloodstream; and muscle cramps, a common affliction in later years, may be caused by a serious lack of this important mineral.

Magnesium, another essential body mineral, is important

for proper relaxation of your muscle tissues. Because of its direct influence on the muscles, liberal amounts of magnesium —either obtained from foods, or in a balanced mineral concentrate—can help prevent the loose, sagging muscles that cause a wrinkled face and neck.

Your old friends the B-vitamins, and pyridoxine in particular, pop up again. This time in connection with your muscles. Dr. Tom Spies was treating a number of patients for pellagra. Because these patients showed further signs of thiamin and riboflavin deficiencies, they were also treated with these B-vitamins.

Yet they still continued to complain of muscular weakness and difficulty in walking—along with nervousness, insomnia, irritability and abdominal pains. Then Dr. Spies decided to add pyridoxine to the treatment. Within twenty-four hours, all signs of muscular weakness and pain had completely disappeared, along with the other unpleasant symptoms. One patient who had been unable to walk more than a few steps prior to being given the pyridoxine treatment *walked two miles* on the same day this vitamin was added to his diet.

Pyridoxine has also been used in treating various types of muscular rigidity, leg stiffness, paralysis and hand tremors. The result has been a marked relief in these unpleasant ailments which all too frequently afflict the past-forty group.

From all these facts you can easily comprehend that the same *planned diet* which will keep your eyes, hair and skin attractively healthy will also help maintain the strength and *youthfulness* of your bones and muscles.

But don't expect to enjoy strong bones or firm muscles on a diet of tea and toast, or rice and gravy. Foods that will give you high proteins, minerals and vitamins are the conditioners that your bones and muscles cry out for continually *at any age.*

Chapter 17

YOUR NERVES MUST STAY YOUNG, TOO

JITTERY nerves in a woman do not please a man, regardless of whatever youthful charms she may possess. Although a young girl, or a woman in her twenties or early thirties, may get by without much poise and with nervous gestures that irritate the onlooker, the older she grows the more these undesirable nervous habits detract from the charm of a woman who wishes to retain an illusion of youth past her fortieth birthday.

Healthy nerves are fully as necessary in a man. Yet I choose to address this chapter directly to you women, although what I say to you holds equally good for the nervous system in past-forty male bodies.

A *planned diet* can give you the healthy nerves so vital to the charm and poise of a lovely woman. Notice, please, that I said a planned diet, and not a "starvation" diet. The nervous system that is starved of protein and fat has no other choice except to become "jittery."

An indifferent diet, or a starvation reducing diet that neglects protein and natural fats, is a diet designed to give you the unwelcome gift of jangled nerves.

Since all women and men past the age of forty must undergo the climacteric with its general disturbance of the endocrine glands and their hormone output (see Chapter 8), liberal amounts of high-protein foods are urgently needed at this time of life to avoid the "middle-aged nerves" which can lessen your personal efficiency and alienate your social world.

Your endocrine glands need high-protein foods to produce their nerve-calming hormones. A disturbance in the thyroid or pituitary glands which commonly attends the menopause may cause a woman to begin gaining weight. This usually makes her all the more eager to adopt the first fad diet that comes her way. Seldom will she stop to question whether her new weight-control regimen contains enough *fat, protein, thiamine* and other *B-vitamins, calcium* and *magnesium* to keep her nerves, glands, muscles and vital organs properly nourished.

And as a result of her woefully substandard diet, she becomes irritable, peevish and jittery. She drives herself and those around her into a frenzy.

I have seen case after case, as have physicians all over the country, of women (a few men, as well) who, after dieting themselves into a critical state of protein-starvation, have turned to cigarettes, alcohol, drugs or sleeping pills to "ease" their tortured nerves.

Diet has a direct, and very important, influence on your nerves and your disposition. Elimination of an important high-protein food from your diet, for no reason other than that it has "too many calories," means depriving your body of several vitally necessary food elements.

To illustrate: the high-protein foods such as cheese, meat, eggs and seed cereals are also rich sources of thiamine (vitamin B-1), known to nutritional science as the "nerve vitamin."

The older you grow, the more thiamine your body needs.

When the diet of any person past forty lacks generous amounts of thiamine, one of the first symptoms is likely to be certain unpleasant changes in disposition. Even the calmest, most amiable person, when seriously starved for thiamine, will become irritable, depressed, suspicious, quarrelsome, jealous and generally neurotic.

Insomnia and extreme sensitivity to noise and trivial vexations will make life a round of petty hells for this thiamine-hungry person.

It may surprise you to learn that a thiamine deficiency can aggravate overweight, since too little of this B-vitamin in the diet leads to a craving for sweets. What irony! The more you crave these forbidden foods, the more irritable your jangled nerves will make you. Instead, why not consider a reducing diet that feeds you too well to permit a sweet craving to make life miserable for you? I've planned such a diet for you in Part II.

I have seen cases where jittery, nerve-jangled men and women of middle age have banished their aging nervous habits and unsocial dispositions almost overnight after their starved nerves began receiving the food elements needed to feed the nervous system.

One such case was that of a woman beautician whose fashionable salon in a large eastern city is frequented each year by hundreds of women in search of their youth. But the proprietress herself, despite the outward care lavished on her own face and body, was *nerve-old* at forty-seven.

To achieve the svelte figure which she advocated to her clientele, she had existed for long periods at a stretch on practically nothing except orange juice, lettuce salads, black coffee and cigarettes.

When I first saw her, she was a creamed and dyed, yet haggard and tense woman whose nervous habits told me that her nerves were starving. Her lack of poise and nerve control made her look a lot older than her forty-seven years.

It took a bit of persuading, since she was abnormally afraid of gaining weight, to "sell" her on the weight-control diet outlined in Part II. She almost demanded a guarantee that she would not begin to "bulge here and there" if she followed this more satisfying diet.

But follow it she finally did, and in a matter of days almost, she began to lose those taut, irritable, fidgety mannerisms which had detracted noticeably from her natural charm.

So successful was her trial of the high-protein reducing diet that it has now become part of the beauty regimen she recommends for her own clientele. And for her common sense, I award her an honorable mention.

If your nervous symptoms indicate the need of extra thiamine in your diet, by all means select a reliable thiamine concentrate, but under no circumstances neglect the foods rich in the B-vitamins. Your body is unable to store large amounts of thiamine, so ample quantities of this B-vitamin must be supplied in the everyday diet.

(Remember also that thiamine is easily destroyed by cooking, and is extremely soluble in water. Foods containing thiamine should be cooked as little as possible, and at low heat, to preserve this nutrient so urgently needed by your nerves.)

A well-planned diet recognizes that certain minerals are also needed to keep the nervous system in first-class working order. *Calcium* and *magnesium* are relaxers for your jangled nerves. The nerves use calcium to transport impulses. When this mineral is not adequately supplied, your nerves can become tense and irritated.

Magnesium has a direct bearing on nerve control. The blood of persons suffering from extreme irritability has been found extremely low in magnesium. This mineral has an important influence on nerve action, and the relaxation of muscle tissues. If you are existing on a diet composed mainly of starchy, devitalized foods, with little or no green vegetables and fresh fruits, the odds are about even that your body needs magnesium.

Because nervousness and lack of self-confidence are outstanding symptoms of the anemia caused by too little *iron* in the body, this mineral is also an essential for good nerves and a poise that attracts.

Another factor in the health of your nervous system is *vitamin D,* perhaps mainly because the calcium in your body may be absorbed more readily when a sufficient amount of the "sunshine vitamin" is present.

We also have learned that when *vitamin A* is scarce enough in the diet to cause eye disorders, an accompanying symptom is a nervousness and general fatigue that interferes with personal contentment and efficiency.

You can scarcely hope to retain the relaxed mannerisms of youth if you allow yourself to become grouchy, uncoöperative, irritable, jittery, tense and quick to anger. These are unpleasant disposition traits that we've come to associate more or less with age—the crotchety old man in the play and the bad-tempered old lady in the novel are stereotyped characters taken from real life.

But if you visualize yourself as a cheerful person, even-tempered in times of stress and excitement, with steady, relaxed nerves that allow you to sleep well, and to meet each day's problems with poise and graciousness, then *you must beware not to let your nerves grow old.*

Chapter 18

YOUR BLOOD CAN MAKE YOU LOOK YOUNGER

WITHOUT blood that is kept *young*—that is, rich with *red* coloring matter—along with the rest of your physical and mental organism, your efforts to remain a radiantly healthy, young-looking person are doomed to failure almost at the outset. For the blood is your body's "carrier system." In order to dispatch *renewed youthfulness* to all other parts of your body, you first must make certain that your carrier system is in A-1 working order.

Since the degree of your natural attractiveness is likewise determined to an important extent by what goes on "behind the skin curtain" covering your body, it would be extremely unwise to slight the bloodstream in your campaign of eating to look younger.

The *cosmetic* effect of healthy blood has never been fully appreciated. It's only when the blood is youthfully red and healthy that it can impart to your body—the outer *you*—all the desirable appearances of a prolonged youth: fresh complexion, naturally red lips and naturally pink fingernails.

How do you keep your blood "youthfully red and healthy"? Mainly through a planned diet—a diet that either cures anemia or prevents your developing it. For anyone may become anemic, at any age; and anemia is the foe of a youthful bloodstream.

In simple language, this is what happens when you are anemic: The salty, straw-colored liquid called blood plasma in which float both red and white blood corpulscles either (1) does not have enough red blood cells, or (2) the red blood cells the plasma does have do not contain enough *hemoglobin*, the red coloring matter that gives blood its rich, red hue.

Hemoglobin is very important in your bloomstream. Some folks think it's the red blood cell itself that is so important, whereas actually it's what the red blood cell *contains*—the hemoglobin, or oxygen-carrying substance in your blood—that causes all the fuss when not present in full force.

And, if we are to "tell all" about the red blood cell, we might as well admit that he is merely a "container"—that is, he exists merely to carry the very important hemoglobin.

(You might be interested to know that the red blood cell is shaped roughly like a doughnut with the hole depressed instead of being punched out; and it's within the spongy, outer rim around the depressed middle that the hemoglobin is carried.)

Without his full quota of hemoglobin, the red blood cell is a pale, colorless, washed-out-looking fellow—about as pallid as the anemic person who does not have enough hemoglobin-filled red blood cells in his arteries.

And this red blood cell is not a very long-lived fellow, either. His average life span is only about thirty days. So your body is continually demanding red blood cell replacements.

Why do we classify hemoglobin as very important? Because this red coloring matter has the top priority job of absorbing oxygen from the lungs, and then distributing it throughout the body to all the cells, picking up carbon dioxide (a waste product from the burning of oxygen in the cells) and carrying this waste gas on the return trip to the lungs where it's expelled from the body in the outgoing breath.

Not exactly an idle fellow, is he, this *hemoglobin* you must be sure to have "enough of"?

When you become anemic, that is, when your body doesn't have enough hemoglobin on the job in your bloodstream, this never-ceasing business of furnishing oxygen to the cells and carrying off their waste products is certain to bog down, much as the food-distribution and garbage-disposal systems of a large city are disrupted when the truck drivers go on a strike.

Very well, if hemoglobin and his container, the red blood cell, are so important to a healthy body, let's feed them their favorite foods.

What are the "favorite foods" of hemoglobin and the red blood cell? Several of the same food elements that also feed your eyes, skin, heart, glands, brain cells—*protein*, the minerals *iron, copper* and *iodine*, and the B-vitamins, especially *thiamine, niacin, pyridoxine, biotin, folic acid* and B-12.

Protein is just as important to the richness of your blood as iron, since the hemoglobin is largely made up of both protein and iron. The red blood cell "containers" that carry the hemoglobin are themselves made of protein. Even a mild deficiency of high proteins in the diet can result in too few of these hemoglobin-carrying cells, as well as too little hemoglobin in the red corpuscles that do exist.

Iron is widely advertised as the mineral responsible for the redness of your blood, and this is true. Yet iron is not the only mineral needed to combat anemia. Copper, too, is necessary before the iron can go to work. Iodine is still another mineral concerned with keeping your blood up to its normal richness. When too little iodine is obtained through your meals, the bone marrow (the red blood cell factory) cannot produce enough red corpuscles, even though both iron and copper are plentiful in the list of minerals essential for "feeding" the blood.

Although men can become anemic the same as women for lack of these food elements in their diets, women are far more susceptible to anemia than men. The reason for this is largely attributable to their periodic loss of blood, without care being taken to restore the valuable supplies of body iron lost each month. Because of this, women require *three to four times* more iron than men during their lifetime.

Again the problem of digestion enters the picture, especially for the person past forty. Since iron dissolves only in acid (the same as protein and calcium can only be digested by acid), it is important to make sure that the hydrochloric acid in your stomach juices is strong enough to handle the iron in the foods you eat. Any foods containing acids, such as buttermilk, sour milk, yogurt, cottage cheese made from soured milk, citrus fruits, apples and other tart fruits, aid the body in absorbing iron.

Regardless of what you've heard for years—that "spinach is full of iron"—this is one vegetable I never recommend. Not only does spinach have a high percentage of oxalic acid (the chemical that combines with calcium in the body to form those excruciatingly painful kidney and bladder stones), but oxalic acid also prevents the iron in spinach from being used by the body since it teams up with the iron to form insoluble compounds. So you may forget all about eating your spinach as far as I'm concerned. Kale is a much better source of food iron than spinach, so if you enjoy cooked greens, you might make a note of this.

The four foods, in order, that produce for you the most hemoglobin are *liver, kidney, apricots* and *egg yolk*.

Even though a food may contain a large percentage of iron,

what's more important to you and your blood is *how much* of that iron is actually available for use in your body.

Meat contains lots of iron, yet not all of it is available for use in the body. For instance, your body can absorb no more than 50 per cent of the iron contained in muscle meats such as lean beef and lamb; 70 per cent of the iron in liver (in spite of the fact that liver produces more hemoglobin than any other known food); and 80 per cent from heart.

This does not mean that meats are not excellent sources of iron, for they most certainly are. What it does mean is that you cannot count on assimilating all the iron listed in a chart as contained in meats.

The average woman needs a *minimum* of 15 milligrams of iron a day to assure her body of an abundance of healthy red blood—more than this if her menstrual flow is heavy. And the average man needs at least 12 milligrams. Since any excess amount of iron in the diet is excreted and can do no harm, the best and safest policy is to obtain too much iron in the daily diet rather than too little.

The menus for your Eat-and-Grow-Younger program, given in Part II, were designed to provide ample quantities of the food elements needed to build and maintain healthy blood. But if your blood has been seriously anemic for a long period, then you may need to take supplemental measures to build it up to normal again.

The apricot tonic given in Chapter 9 may be all that's needed to create a maximum of hemoglobin in your blood, or you may still require supplemental doses of a good mineral concentrate containing iron.

Remember to take care of your red blood cells and the precious *red* hemoglobin contained in them, and they, in turn, will take care of the radiant appearance associated with youth. Healthy blood, teeming with hemoglobin-laden red corpuscles, is one cosmetic you cannot buy at a counter.

Chapter 19

YOUTH BEGINS AT BREAKFAST

For years you've been assured that "life begins at forty." And so it does—if your middle years are protected from the serious ailments that often sneak in with the fortieth birthday.

But I doubt if you've given much thought to the fact that *youth begins at breakfast*.

I consider breakfast the most important meal of the day. For me it is always a high-protein meal, with little or no pure starch of any kind. Nor is this merely a whim of mine. There's a solid nutritional basis for eating high-protein breakfasts, and eliminating the pure starches from your "wake-up" meal.

My breakfast menu sometimes causes comment among my fellow breakfasters whenever I am away from home.

I remember one morning in the dining room of a Pittsburgh hotel when I ordered sliced oranges, two broiled lamb chops, and a cube of cheese for my breakfast. The waitress repeated the order as though I had ordered hummingbird tongues, then set off doubtfully toward the kitchen.

At that particular time I was just beginning a series of difficult lectures, all the while trying to rush to completion the manuscript of one of my earlier books. I needed all the energy I could muster—and I knew that *each day's energy is supplied primarily at breakfast*.

But the weary-looking couple at the table next to mine evidently didn't agree with my choice of breakfast. For, as the waitress placed the platter of nicely browned chops in front of me, I heard the woman murmur to her husband, "Disgusting! A regular cannibal's breakfast." And then she and her husband smugly downed their own all-starch breakfast of a patented dry cereal, sweet roll and coffee.

Yet I'll wager that around eleven o'clock that morning I had by far the more energetic body, and the best-controlled nerves of the three. And all because I had the foresight to supply my mind and body with the type of food—*high-protein*—that assures the most nourishment for muscles, nerves and brain cells.

Although you may not have realized it, your disposition— your "mood," that is—for the day is largely determined by the kind of breakfast you eat. A high-starch breakfast starts you out for the day with your appetite temporarily appeased, yet with your digestive tract laboring under the burden of a lot of gooey food that probably will have you belching before you leave the table.

As the gas from this undigested starchy mass accumulates in your digestive tract, crowding uncomfortably around your heart, you begin feeling as though you shouldn't have gotten out of bed at all that morning. Your night's rest apparently did you little good, for you are tired and weary even before the morning gets well under way.

Show me where the average high-starch breakfast of fruit

juice, white toast, devitalized cereal and white-sugared coffee contains any *thiamine* to feed hard-working nerves and brain cells, and I'll be glad to give up my own high-protein, thiamine-containing breakfasts of meat, eggs, fish, cheese and seed cereals.

But, until such proof is forthcoming (and I'm safe in making this offer, because "proof" of this erroneous nutritional fact can never be made), I shall continue eating the highly proteinized breakfasts that I know are teeming with the energy I shall require to perform each day's tasks to the best of my ability—to say nothing of fortifying me against succumbing to the irritations of the hundred and one little things that constantly arise to try one's patience.

Day after day of breakfasts low in high-protein and thiamine-rich foods are responsible for more than half the supersensitive, depressed, quarrelsome, non-cooperative people in this country. And I hesitate to estimate how much domestic unhappiness traces back to breakfasts that fail to prepare bodies and minds for the give-and-take of everyday living in our nerve-trying era.

Most high-protein foods are rich in thiamine, particularly egg yolk, lean beef and lamb, and seed cereals such as millet and sunflower seed.

A splendid *energy breakfast* is one consisting of fruit (whole or sliced citrus fruits, not the juice alone, melon, berries, pineapple or other fresh or sun-dried fruits), scrambled eggs to which dry skim milk powder and grated cheese have been added for flavor and extra protein, served with hot millet meal mush cooked in liquid milk made from the powdered skim milk and served with honey.

A light breakfast of fruit juice, toast and coffee is not sufficient nourishment to carry the hungry body (remember, you've not eaten for nearly twelve hours when you sit down to the breakfast table) through a morning's work with full vigor and efficiency. The word breakfast means exactly that —"break the fast."

The business of skipping breakfast entirely is an extremely foolish habit for anyone, but more particularly so for the person who wants to encourage his body to remain youthfully strong and vigorous. Many women—men, too—entertain the false idea that by skipping breakfast they will "lose weight."

This reminds me of the nearing-forty wife of a friend of mine. A devotee of the "I must diet" cult, she religiously skips her breakfast every morning, momentarily quieting her rumbling stomach with several cups of strong black coffee and a cigarette or two.

But along about ten o'clock she is forced to succumb to those persistent hunger pangs which were not appeased by the black-coffee-and-cigarette breakfast. One or two white-bread sandwiches are washed down, either by a soft drink from the refrigerator or by more coffee, and topped off by a wedge of pie or a slice of cake left over from a previous meal.

She reconciles herself to the number of calories in this high-starch snack with the thought that she "saved a lot of calories" by not eating breakfast.

I need not explain that this haphazard dieter does not lose weight. Nor do I need to tell you that she is a highly nervous, often unreasonable woman who looks at least a good five years more than her real age.

A series of studies undertaken at the University of Iowa College of Medicine brought out some startling facts about breakfast-skippers that caused the doctors making the study to issue this warning: *Not eating breakfast is both unwise and harmful.*

The women volunteers, who did without their breakfasts for the purposes of this dietetic survey, showed a marked drop in their working efficiency. Their reactions were decidedly slowed down. And a marked increase was noted in their neuro-muscular tremors. This means that they could not work as well, or as untiringly; they were more likely to meet with accidents because of their slowed-down reactions, and their nervous and muscular control fell way below normal.

The men taking part in this experiment showed the same harmful effects, only more so. They complained more about being hungry, and experienced greater fatigue after strenuous exercise. A few of the men even complained of dizziness and nausea.

I hope that the unthinking wives who send their husbands out to work each morning without breakfast, or with a hastily thrown together affair of coffee, toast and dry cereal, will ponder awhile on the foregoing paragraph.

If your husband is showing signs of "slipping," might not the cause lie in your own failure to send him forth nutritionally well prepared each morning for the day's physical and mental strains?

Such wives might also give thought to the fact that the same kind of inadequate breakfasts which age their husbands also cause the years to be unkind to them.

It's very pleasant, I realize, to lie in bed until the very last minute, and then make a dash for the kitchen, set the coffee perking, throw a couple slices of white bread into the automatic toaster, and pour some dry cereal from the package into a bowl at each place.

But the time "saved" by such nutritionally unsafe breakfasts is piling up for you and for your family—piling up in the unwanted premature aging that is lurking around the corner to overtake you along about the fortieth birthday. Or to hasten a natural advance in years into a crippled senility.

Everyone, no matter what their present age, needs the irreplaceable nutrition provided by a high-protein breakfast for a body that has been fasting all night long.

If you can afford meat only once a day, I would be inclined to advise you to enjoy this splendid high-protein food at breakfast—a leisurely breakfast that you've given yourself time enough to eat in comfort by arising an hour earlier than usual.

A typical breakfast in the Argentine is simply a piece of pan-broiled steak served with an egg. I discovered that this is the favorite breakfast or luncheon dish of the hardy Argentine working man and woman in the cities of Buenos Aires and Rosario. And I might add that it has become one of my favorites, too—a dish that followed me home to be added to our list of high-protein breakfast dishes.

A high-protein breakfast may be a radical departure from your present eating habits. But you must remember one thing: *Your day can be no better than the foundation laid for that day.* And your breakfast is the *nutritional foundation* you lay each morning for the activities of the next twelve to sixteen hours.

If you lack pep, are always just one step ahead of collapsing into a chair, and never can quite get around to finishing your work, change to a high-protein breakfast. You'll amaze yourself by how quickly you begin perking up.

Here are a few general suggestions. (Breakfast menus and recipes are given in Part II.) First, take your time while eating breakfast, even if it means getting up thirty minutes or an hour earlier. You cannot get the maximum good out of your breakfast, or any meal for that matter, if your mind is racing away from the table. Relax, enjoy your food and let your stomach have at least half an hour for full concentration on its job before you go dashing off on the day's round of activities.

Eat all the fresh fruit you want at breakfast, preferably the *whole* fruit. Fruit is a pleasant food with which to begin any meal, and is an excellent way of preparing the stomach for the other food to follow. Drink whatever beverage you like —only don't dump the contents of the sugar bowl into it.

If you like your morning cup of coffee or tea sweetened, for a real energy beverage try honey instead of white sugar. The spoonful or so of honey you use will, in itself, be a splendid energizer.

But whatever fruit, beverage, or high-protein dish you choose for breakfast, no pure-starch foods. No white-bread toast, no sweet rolls, no devitalized cereals. (And don't be tempted into sneaking a piece of toast or a roll merely because no one is looking. Someone *is* watching you—the vision of the youthful person you want to be.)

The worst breakfast-time sinner of all is the person who takes only a cup of black coffee. He commits the unforgivable sin of stimulating his body while denying it the nourishment demanded by such stimulation.

You cannot expect a hasty, ill-planned breakfast and a quick, equally protein-deficient lunch to keep your body fueled and energized throughout the very hours of the day when you put the greatest strain on your nerves, brain cells and muscles.

This habit of saving up all day for a heavy meal at night is what puts the "spare tire" around the waistline.

Experiments conducted at the University of Chicago have disclosed that the food eaten at an evening dinner is transformed mainly into fat, and not into useful energy. Because you go to bed shortly after that heavy evening meal, your body does not require the energy it does throughout your long waking hours.

And for that reason the food consumed at this late meal is stored rather than burned.

Stored, I must warn you, as fat deposits in the liver, around the heart and in the arteries.

This explains why I teach that your breakfasts should be full meals, not stop-gap, hastily snatched snacks. And your evening meal should be a light one—although nutritious—so that the unburned energy foods eaten at that later hour are not allowed to store up overnight as unwanted fat around the waistline, or in most dangerous of all places—the arteries.

Proteinize your breakfasts for energy without stuffiness. Smaller amounts of food, if that food is high-protein, satisfy the appetite without the bulk of a carbohydrate meal necessary to quiet hunger pangs.

I guarantee you that a breakfast, say, of two scrambled eggs (boiled, poached, coddled or shirred are equally nutritious), a cube of cheese or a portion of cottage cheese, plus whatever fruit and beverage you prefer, will leave you far more satisfied, with absolutely no sense of being stuffed, than if you had eaten enough of a high-starch breakfast to satisfy your hunger.

Now about your lunch—instead of spaghetti, baked macaroni, or a sandwich and a piece of pie, fortify your mind and body for the balance of its day's work by choosing a dish containing another high-protein food—meat, fish, poultry, cheese or a good meat substitute made from whole seed cereals as explained in Part II. Add to this a vegetable or a green salad, top it off with a light fruit or custard dessert, and you have the perfect, pep-supplying luncheon.

What's more, by the time evening comes, you'll find that your appetite isn't so ravenous that it demands the accustomed heavy dinner. Another light protein-vegetable-and-fruit meal will be all your appetite demands; and most certainly you'll sleep far better, and wake up the next morning more refreshed than if your body had struggled all night through the digestion of a heavy, high-starch dinner.

You'll feel—and look—younger. Your figure will become trimmer. Your muscles firmer. Your step lighter. Your working capacity greater. Your vigor more pronounced.

The time to begin dealing knockout punches to a premature old age is at breakfast!

Chapter 20

WHAT ABOUT FOOD COMBINATIONS?

WHENEVER I'm asked about "food combinations"—which is frequently—I feel like the old country doctor who was asked by an anxious young mother whether castor oil was good for her child. To which the old doctor replied: "If you can get it down him, it is. If you can't, it isn't!"

If a food combination is good nutrition, it's all right. If it's not, it isn't!

Let's start out with an *all-protein diet*—the simplest possible diet, composed of the one food element capable of supporting the body in radiant health.

In the spring of 1906, the now world-famous Vilhjalmur Stefansson made his first trip to the Arctic as the anthropologist of a polar expedition. Six months later, through a series of unforeseen events, he found himself separated from the rest of the expedition, and forced to live for a year with the Eskimos in the far northern part of Canada.

During all the time of his enforced stay with these people of the Far North, Stefansson's diet consisted of protein-meat (mostly caribou or seal), meat broth and fish eaten with whale oil. No salt, no bread, no vegetables, or fruit—nothing but meat and fish. An all-protein diet.

At first, he only nibbled at the fresh salmon roasted specially for him (the Eskimos eat their fish boiled). In his diary he wrote "what a terrible time" he was having. But after several weeks, much to his surprise, he found himself enjoying the boiled salmon along with his Eskimo hosts; and he would tear into a chunk of caribou meat with the same zest with which he formerly had tackled a porterhouse steak.

The following spring, after six months of this meat-and-fish diet, Stefansson visited a whaling vessel some 200 miles away, and enjoyed New England cooking for a few days. But after this "fling," he returned wholly without regret to his Eskimo diet of meat and fish. Not only that, but he discovered his health couldn't be better, and he was full of an unaccustomed energy while living on this all-protein diet which, contrary to his expectations, did not prove at all monotonous. For, as he expressed it: "You never become tired of your food if you have only one thing to eat."

Nor was this experience on an all-protein diet unique with Stefansson, since he found that the white men he took with him on later polar expeditions also thrived on an exclusively meat-and-fish diet.

This dietary experience prompted Stefansson many years later to volunteer for an all-meat diet experiment at a New York hospital. An experiment, by the way, that caused distinguished American and European physiologists to make flat predictions that the two subjects (Stefansson and a young Dane named Andersen who had been on one of the Arctic expeditions) would not be able to hold out any longer than from three to four days to an outside of three weeks. In fact, one of the most distinguished of the doctors made the statement that he found it easier to believe that Stefansson and the members of his expeditions were "lying" than to believe that they had remained "healthy" for several *years* on an exclusive diet of meat and fish.

Thus it was with a great deal of personal satisfaction that Stefansson and Andersen, both hale and hearty, ended their *twelve months* of living on nothing but meat and fish. In Stefansson's case, however, an exception had been made to include milk products and eggs (all of them high-grade proteins, of course) because he was lecturing throughout the country during that year, and it was not always possible for him to obtain meat or fish for his off-hour meals. But Andersen tasted nothing but meat (that included poultry) and fish for the entire twelve months.

There was no denying the evidence presented in the healthy bodies of these two determined subjects. Both ended the year of their all-protein diets with better health than when they had started it. Moreover, Stefansson, who had been declared ten pounds overweight at the beginning of the year, had lost those unwanted ten pounds soon after beginning the diet, and had then maintained his ideal weight without further difficulty.

In Andersen's case, he had been cured of a tendency to suffer one head cold after another, as had been the case when he began the experiment. He also had been troubled with an intestinal toxemia which had cleared up by the end of the year on the all-protein diet.

This remarkable experiment—which was recorded at length in the medical and nutrition journals—is not recited here to stampede you into a hasty change-over to an all-meat diet. For one thing, you would probably find it too expensive to consume the six pounds of meat, or more, which Stefansson estimated he and Andersen ate each day. But here is the irrefutable answer to the outmoded belief that "too much meat is bad for you"; that it "causes" arthritis, high blood pressure, kidney disorders, hardening of the arteries, even diabetes.

Incidentally, despite the lifelong subjection of the Eskimos to violent extremes in temperature (from the sweltering heat of their igloos to the way-below-zero temperature of outdoors), Stefansson reported having found no rheumatism or arthritis among the Eskimos with whom he lived. Neither did they have decayed teeth, head colds, pneumonia, hardening of the arteries, diabetes or diseased kidneys. All of which should give us pause for thought.

Regardless of any dietary or religious prejudices you may have against eating flesh foods (meats, fish, poultry, eggs, cheese and non-fat milk) the fact remains that they are truly man's "elixir of life"—his pep tonic, his youth-restorer, all combined in one!

In planning your Eat-and-Grow-Younger diet of high-protein foods, I have tried to keep in mind the only important nutritional *taboos* which have a basis in scientific fact:

1. Never combine high-proteins (red meats, poultry, fish, eggs, cheese, milk) with high-starches (rice, macaroni, spaghetti, white bread, rich desserts) at the same meal. And if, for some valid reason, you are forced to eat more high-starch meals than high-protein, then by all means take

liberal amounts of concentrated B-vitamins, since the more starch you eat, the more your body requires the B-complex factors that have the specific task of postponing the day when you must take your final farewell of youth.

2. Avoid combining pure fats with high starches in the same meal. For instance, bacon (almost 100 per cent fat, and of the wrong kind, too), fried potatoes, cream, white sugar, white bread and jelly are a rather common breakfast menu in some homes, yet nothing could be worse nutrition.

It's absolutely impossible to plan a meal that doesn't include some carbohydrate with its proteins; or some fat with its carbohydrate. But the thing to keep in mind is this:

A meal should be predominantly either *protein* or *carbohydrate*. And when it is predominantly protein, it should include only those *natural* starches found in vegetables, fruits, milk and honey or raw sugar. This means, as one example, omitting a rice or macaroni dish and pie with your steaks, substituting the carbohydrates to be found in a green salad, a cooked vegetable and a fruit or custard dessert.

This is a good place to clear the lowly white potato of the many unfounded dietary crimes charged against it. Potatoes, either baked or steamed in the skin, are a good food and do *not* come under the heading of the starches to be omitted from a protein meal. Forget all those things you've heard about "cutting out potatoes because they make you fat." It's not the potato that adds the calories, but the grease it's fried in, or the gravies poured over it.

There are sound physiological reasons behind the two "food combination" taboos given above.

Nature has provided each human body with two separate digestive processes—an *acid* process for digesting proteins, and an *alkaline* process for carbohydrates.

Proteins, as explained in an earlier chapter, are digested principally in the stomach by the gastric juices which normally are strongly acid in the healthy stomach, containing as the most important of their ingredients free *hydrochloric acid*.

Carbohydrates—the sugar-and-starch foods—are not digested in the stomach. They receive their processing in the small intestine from alkaline digestive juices which consist mainly of secretions from the pancreas.

This is what happens when your stomach, secreting its acid juices to digest proteins, is also presented with a load of high-starch food at the same time:

The carbohydrates automatically restrict the secretion of

the acid stomach juices, since your very sensitive stomach divines that starch is on the way down, and starch is definitely not its business. This load of starch food, after it reaches the stomach, also combines with some of the already secreted hydrochloric acid that was intended for the protein foods, and carries the acid on into the small intestine, thus depriving the half-digested protein of the acid needed to finish the job.

Not only that, but the introduction of this "stolen" acid into the intestine, where all is supposed to be *alkaline* for processing starches, upsets the balance of the pancreatic hormones and enzymes intended to digest the starchy food.

This fact was developed some years ago in a study conducted at the Mayo Clinic.

When you eat high starches with your high-protein meal, you interrupt the digestion of both types of foods. As a result, you lose the maximum nourishment you should obtain from protein foods, and you burden the intestinal tract with an improperly digested meal.

As for the other nutritional taboo, this is why *pure fats* and *high starches* are incompatible in the same meal.

Fats are intended to leave the stomach, undigested, and pass into the upper intestine where the gall bladder empties its bile to digest them. During this process of digesting fats, certain fatty *acids* are produced which immediately neutralize any alkaline secretions that have been called forth to digest starch foods. The one substance which splits the starch molecule and permits its complete digestion is called *amylopsin* —and amylopsin can work only in an *alkaline* solution.

Therefore, when the fatty acids produced by digestion of pure fat foods are present in the upper intestine at the same time as the alkaline pancreatic secretions, the digestive fluids become neutralized, and amylopsin immediately stops working. This leaves the starch foods only partially digested—and that means gas pains, belching and constipation.

Nature makes combinations of food elements that we should be wise to heed. Fat and protein are found in combination such as the fat in meat, and the cream (fat) and protein in milk. But nowhere in nature will you find pure fat combined with a high-starch food. Consequently, nature did not provide us with a digestive mechanism capable of digesting pure fats and high starches at the same time.

But you won't need to worry over much about "food combinations," if you follow these simple rules which are worked out for you in the menus and recipes given in Part II:

1. Build at least two meals a day around a high-protein

food—red meat, gland and organ meats, fish, poultry, eggs, cheese or seed cereals—combined with fresh salad, vegetables, a cooked vegetable or two and fruits either fresh or cooked. This is the safest food combination to follow, because it not only allows the two digestive processes to function properly, but also because it assures you a regular intake of essential proteins, minerals, and vitamins.

2. When you use cereals and breads, choose only those which will also provide a certain amount of protein, minerals and vitamins, such as whole grains and the seed cereals (millet, sunflower seed, sesame seed).

3. Eat oil-dressed salads with your protein meals, since fats make a good combination with proteins.

4. Use only acid beverages with a protein meal—buttermilk, citrus juices—since *sweet* milk drunk in any quantity with a protein meal neutralizes the acid stomach juices. This applies to plain sweet milk, cocoa, hot chocolate, milk shakes and malted milks. Of course, tea or coffee may be taken after any meal.

5. The time for that "one per cent dissipation" on sweets you're allowed is either *between meals,* or with a high-starch meal—never with a high-protein meal.

I have always hesitated to dwell at length on "food combinations" in my lectures because of the possibility that I might be misunderstood, thereby becoming the unwitting cause of creating another food "faddist."

My advice to you is: *Be sensible, not a faddist.* Don't adopt "food combinations" that violate all the rules of good nutrition and human physiology. Your hold on youth depends on facts, not fads.

Chapter 21

EATING HABITS FOR A LONGER LIFE

"To be happy we must be true to nature and carry our age along with us." You'll notice that the author of this apt quotation did not say "drag," he said *carry.* The years are a "drag" on you only if you are ill, whether ailing with some particular malady or maladies, or only half-sick—not well enough to feel good, yet not quite sick enough to go to bed.

Nutritional scientists, along with the biochemists, are proving more conclusively every day that *most of your ills have their beginnings in poor eating habits.*

If you want to carry your years lightly toward a longer, happier life, rather than allow the years to drag you along through a miserable ailing premature old age you must take time to analyze your current eating habits. Compare them, one by one, with the stay-young dietary habits that make for a stronger, younger-looking, more vigorous *you.*

MAKE PLANNED DIET A HABIT

The kind and quantity of food you eat are largely a matter of habits formed in early childhood. This often explains why obesity runs in certain families, although the fatties may try to explain away their overweight by blaming it on an "inherited family trait." Usually the tendency toward obesity lies, instead, in a common family habit of indulging in large meals of rich, starchy foods. Similarly, the persons who "don't like" this, that or the other food are merely following some childhood eating habit.

From the age of thirty onward, if you value your health, good looks and ability to live a long and vigorous life, *you must change your eating habits.*

The high-energy carbohydrate foods that were tolerated during your earlier years now slow you down and build up deposits of fat in dangerous places. After the super-active childhood years, the exhausting teens and the procreative twenties, few of us are called upon to expend the same amount of energy for daily survival as did our more primitive ancestors. Yet many people go on eating a lumberjack's diet while doing work no more strenuous than sitting at a desk for a few hours a day, or performing a few modernized and mechanized household duties.

After the age of thirty, preferably, and most certainly after forty, you must begin taking stock of your eating habits.

This means *more protein* and vitamin-rich *fruits and vegetables.* And less—perhaps none at all—high-starch foods such as rich desserts, all-starch items like white rice and macaroni, fattening bonbons, highly sugared and carbonated soft drinks, or overindulgence in alcoholic beverages.

This menu-in-a-nutshell is your first and most important step toward the goal of a longer life and a younger-looking body. From now on you must accustom yourself to topping off a meal with fruits (or the permissible desserts given in

Part II) rather than with the rich pastries, cakes, candies and jellies you have formed a habit of expecting at the end of every meal. One of the best means of keeping your sweet tooth under control is by looking to honey (see Chapter 12), nature's own confection, and the only sweet food, besides fruits, that contains valuable food elements.

Bad food habits at any time, and especially during the years that subject men and women to the ordeal of their climacteric (change of life), may be the underlying cause of a physical and mental breakup that can devastate any remnants of youthfulness left to them.

A pitiful case came to my attention several years ago of a forty-nine-year-old woman whose husband had died two years previously, leaving her a childless widow. Since his death, partly because of her grief, but mostly because of the physical inertia resulting from an abnormal menopause, she had not taken the trouble to prepare well-balanced meals for herself. Whenever she felt hungry she existed mainly on easy-to-fix sandwiches, cakes and pies from the bakery, and endless boxes of candy. At the time I first heard of her case, she had sunk into a wretched state of melancholia, sleeplessness, heart palpitation, breathlessness and aching fatigue that had driven her to the border line of insanity.

Under the watchful eye of her sister who lived in the same city, this middle-aged widow was put on an emergency vitamin treatment to counteract the serious dietary deficiencies resulting from two years of these ruinous eating habits. And she was made to eat meals that began at breakfast with high-protein foods such as meat, eggs, cheese, fish, or seed cereals; continuing with more protein foods for lunch; and ending up the day with yet another protein meal, light but nourishing, of millet or sunflower seed served with non-fat milk, a cube of cheese and a dish of fruit.

For a mid-morning energizer, she was taught to drink a large cup of warmed milk (made extra protein-rich by mixing one tablespoon of powdered skim milk with one cup of water) flavored with a teaspoon of honey. Her afternoon snack was usually a cup of tea (sometimes the aromatic herb tea brewed from fenugreek seeds and flavored with honey), served with a few seed-cakes or several pieces of fruit dainties (see Part II).

Within three months' time, this woman had made so dramatic a recovery from her mental and physical breakdown that she was able to obtain, and hold, a responsible position with a large welfare organization. Because of her reformed eating habits, she was also able to pass through the remainder of her menopause with no undue discomfort—and today she looks *younger* than she did at the time her husband died.

Nor are middle-aged women the only violators of good eating habits. Many men are such prejudiced eaters (usually it's the wife or mother who "spoils" them by catering to their prejudices) that they deliberately slight the foods most needed by their older bodies at a time when mind, muscles, nerves and sex glands are undergoing a period of readjustment similar to the menopause experienced by a woman.

You can be unwise at the table during your teens and your earlier years, and still get by, but your eating sins will come home to roost if you persist in following youth-destroying food habits past the age of forty.

Let me repeat: The matter of food likes—and dislikes—is largely a matter of habit. Therefore, train yourself to *like* the foods that do the most toward preserving your youth and fortifying you against an early and a senile old age. For example, instead of thinking, "But I don't like cheese," start thinking for a change, "I want to feel and look younger, and cheese is a protein food that can help my body accomplish this goal."

With this kind of positive thought, it won't be long before your taste buds will develop a real appreciation for the subtle flavors to be found in the different kinds of cheeses—in other protein and natural foods, too. Make these your *first foods* in every meal, because they are the foods that can help you look and feel younger.

If you want your "body's worth" from the meals you eat, that is, if you are eager to regain the appearances and sensations of a youthful body, then you must acquire the *habit* of a high-protein, planned diet. Oh, I'm not saying that an occasional variation will do you too much harm. But don't count on these periodic diet dissipations to supply you with that day's needed quota of protein, minerals and vitamins.

DIGESTIVE AIDS NOT FOUND IN DRUGSTORES

Another habit that will contribute to your health and long "youth" is that of aiding your middle-aged stomach to do a thorough job of digesting the proteins you eat.

As explained in the preceding chapter, digesting protein food is the main job of your stomach (carbohydrates and fats, except milk fat, are processed in the upper intestinal tract). And to break down the proteins you eat into the amino acids which are the only forms of protein that can be carried by your bloodstream, nature has provided your stomach with digestive juices that normally are strong acids. These acid stomach juices, when strong enough, reduce all protein foods to a pulpy mass. The fibers of that steak you eat, when properly digested, should become as liquefied as though the meat had been pulverized in a powerful grinder and mixed with water.

Not only is the hydrochloric acid in your stomach juices an effective pulverizer, it is also a powerful germ-killer. As an experiment, you might place a little chopped meat in a glass of water and let it stand in a warm place. Before long, the contents will start to putrefy rapidly.

But now place a little hydrochloric acid in another glass of water, add some more chopped meat, and repeat the experiment. This time you'll notice that no putrefaction sets in, because the acid destroys the germs and fungi which cling to all food, regardless of the care with which it is handled.

Likewise, when your stomach is healthy—that is, when its juices are strongly acid—your food digests instead of putrefying. Ordinarily, the billions of bacteria and fungi that get into your stomach each day fall into a strong acid bath and are destroyed. But if your stomach acids are not potent enough to kill these invaders, or to do a thorough job of pulverizing your protein foods, you may be headed for trouble—the kind of trouble that makes you feel ill, dispirited and too "old" to get the most out of life.

As though all this weren't enough, I should warn you also that no matter how conscientiously you attempt to follow the high-protein diet regimen outlined in this book, it will do little good toward making you look and feel younger *if your stomach acids are too weak* to properly digest the protein foods you eat. For this reason, it behooves you to make certain that strong digestive juices await the food you send into your stomach.

There are several ways to stimulate your stomach cells into secreting digestive juices that are strongly acid. Pleasant ways, I might add—ways that have been largely overlooked in our American eat-on-the-run meals.

Start your meals with fruit, a cup of vegetable soup, a bouillon or a meat broth. Why? Because fresh fruits and their juices (dry wines, also) and the extracted juices of vegetables, together with meat extract or the bouillon made by simmering meats and vegetables together, are rich in certain *extractive substances*. When these foods reach the stomach before a meal, their extractive substances cause certain groups of cells in your lower stomach to produce a hormone known as *secretin* that passes directly into the bloodstream and is carried to all the organs, including the glands in the upper section of the stomach. Here the *secretin* hormone excites the gastric glands into producing and pouring forth into the stomach large amounts of the very powerful hydrochloric acid which is absolutely essential for thorough digestion of a protein meal.

European and Oriental eating habits have made use of this important digestive secret for centuries. Broths and dry wines are everyday mealtime accessories. Rarely do you find a European home where the family sits down and immediately dives into the entree or main course. Step by step, the stomach is encouraged to prepare for its main digestive task through the sipping of dry wines, and the spooning of light broths.

If you have no prejudice against it, a very small glass of a low-alcohol dry wine sipped before the meal can be a valuable aid to digestion in persons past forty. However, please don't get the idea that I am advocating the use of liquor, for I am violently opposed to alcoholism and all that it represents. But the light 12-per-cent—or less—wines to be found on European and South American tables are far from being intoxicating. In fact, after a vintage year (a year when the grape develops a great deal of sugar and the alcoholic content of the wine runs high), the wine makers dilute their dry wines with water to make them appropriate for table use.

Remember, though, that cocktails and highballs are *not* digestive aids, to be used the same as a very low-alcohol dry wine, because they do not contain the extractive substances from fruit, and because their alcoholic content runs too high. About the best these dubious beverages can do for you is to give you a dizzy head, and add calories to your daily quota.

I have even hesitated to mention dry wines as a digestive aid for fear of providing a ready-made excuse for some intemperate person to indulge his or her weakness. So let me repeat:

The *dry* table wine, to be taken solely as a digestive aid, must be used in very small quantities and must be a low-alcohol wine, that is, 12-per-cent or less. If you cannot find one with that little alcohol, buy a good dry wine, and dilute it yourself with about two parts wine to one part water. Actually, some of our medicinal preparations contain more alcohol than a European table wine.

In recent years, we have learned that the vitamins of the B-complex group, particularly *thiamine,* are needed by the stomach for producing its digestive acids. From this you can quickly grasp why the average devitalized, high-starch, low-vitamin diet is the prime cause of our national maladies—*indigestion* and *constipation.*

There is yet another "homemade" remedy for good digestion. Do you try to *keep happy at mealtime?* If not, you are placing a burden on your stomach glands so onerous that poor digestion is the inevitable result.

The glands in your stomach (as well as the salivary glands in your mouth) are stimulated into action by your desire for food; by the sight, smell and taste of appetizing food; and by the *calmness* of your emotional state. Very often the thoughts in your mind, and the emotions produced by those thoughts, have a greater influence on the acidity and quantity of your digestive juices than does the food you eat.

One disturbing or irritating thought is all it takes to put the brakes on your digestive machinery. Distressing news, angry words, nauseating subjects or the sight of unappetizing food prevent you from digesting your meal, whether or not you think you are "sensitive" to such mealtime unpleasantness.

A meal that is going to be thoroughly digested and assimilated into the bloodstream (the first and only place where your food can begin its work of nourishing the body cells) is the meal that is eaten without any emotional disturbance. *Good spirits are essential for proper digestion.*

After you master the *art of eating,* along with the art of planning your meals, you will have taken another long stride toward your goal of a longer life, and a healthier one.

And for the sake of your confused stomach, throw away those "alkalizer" tablets and powders that do nothing except make you burp a little, all the while they are decreasing the acidity of a stomach which already contains *too little acid* for good digestion. Such "remedies" profit no one except their manufacturers.

This is a timely spot to bring up the subject of *chewing.* A lot of false information and erroneous advice has been handed out to the public for years on the subject of "proper mastication of food." Once and for all, I would like to clear up these mistaken ideas, and present the true facts. In brief, here is your "chewing chart":

1. *All vegetables, fruits and sugar-starch foods should be chewed thoroughly.* Carbohydrates are digested in an alkaline base, as I've explained before. The saliva in your mouth is an alkali, and is secreted by the salivary glands as the first step in the long and complicated digestion of carbohydrates. Therefore, if you bolt your carbohydrate foods, you cause them to miss this preliminary digestive processing, with the end result that they reach the upper intestinal tract (where the processing is completed) inadequately prepared for the final steps. All herbivorous

animals, such as the cow, rabbit and horse are noted for their long and patient chewing. In so doing, they are following the rules of nature—thorough mastication for carbohydrates in order to mix them well with the alkaline saliva of the mouth.

2. *All protein foods such as meat, fish, poultry, eggs and cheese require little chewing for good digestion.* No doubt this comes as a surprise to you—a complete reversal of everything you've ever been taught about mastication. Meat has been conscientiously and laboriously ground for the person with poor, or no, teeth; while eggs have been boiled only enough to set the white for the person with a "weak digestion." All of which has been a serious digestive and nutritional mistake! From recent experiments, some of them conducted at the Mayo Clinic, we now have learned that protein foods which reach the stomach in solid, larger bites will be digested—and assimilated—far better than the ground, soft-cooked or thoroughly masticated proteins.

During the experiment at the Mayo Clinic, it was discovered that meat fed in good-sized bites was digested far better than ground meat. You have only to consider the dog or the lion, both carnivorous, to realize that you've never seen either of these animals patiently masticating their meat as a cow does her cud. For one thing, nature has not given the carnivorous animals teeth for long chewing. Rather, they have been provided teeth for tearing off chunks of a size for convenient swallowing. The dog—and you—can safely swallow protein foods with little chewing because the real work of digesting these proteins is done by the stomach acids. And let me assure you that the hydrochloric acid in your stomach can do a far more thorough job of pulverizing meat fibers than your teeth could ever accomplish.

The fact of the matter is that you actually *waste* protein food by sending it to the stomach in a finely ground, or semi-liquid condition. Why? Because the little valve (pylorus) at the bottom of the stomach is hair-triggered to open and empty the stomach contents into the upper intestine whenever the mass reaches a certain pulpy state. Therefore, a soft-boiled egg will leave the stomach before it is completely broken down by the digestive acids into the amino acids which are used to rebuild body protein. In like manner, ground meats are too quickly liquefied to be completely broken up into their amino acids. So, instead of being assimilated into the bloodstream, much of this partially digested protein is excreted from the body.

This is a good place to pass on to you a bit of wisdom regarding whole fruit versus fruit juices.

I deplore the custom of serving squeezed citrus juices instead of the whole fruit. All fruits (vegetables, too) are carbohydrates. That means their digestion begins *in the mouth*. With that fact in mind, will someone please tell me how you can *chew* a glass of orange juice? The answer, of course, is that you can't. The juice, with its naturally high sugar content, passes immediately through the mouth and stomach, reaching the upper intestine without any predigestion whatsoever.

That is why many of you may have noticed your morning glass of orange juice has a tendency to make you belch, or to cause those "rolling gas pains" in the abdomen. Like all other half-digested carbohydrates, your orange juice begins to ferment in your intestinal tract, sending off gases that cause discomfort. However, had you eaten your breakfast orange, pulp and all, you would have been forced to chew the tough fibers of the whole fruit long enough so that the saliva—a digestive juice—would have been well mixed through it. And by the time the fruit pulp reached the upper intestine, the final digestive processing could have gotten under way with no trouble at all.

Furthermore, the vitamins and minerals of this valuable citrus fruit would have been more completely assimilated into your bloodstream along with the correctly digested mass, instead of being partly lost from the body in the incompletely digested juice.

With fruit juice, there is also the tendency to overindulge. Rarely can you relish more than one whole orange at a time, whereas a thirsty person can easily gulp down a pint, or more, of orange juice. This is too much fruit sugar to reach the upper intestinal tract at one time, without any predigesting by the saliva.

Colitis patients have been advised for years to "eat only *whole* fruits and vegetables." The fermentation gases from incompletely digested fruit and vegetable juices are simply that much added torture to the already irritated intestinal tract of a colitis patient. Yet these same persons can enjoy whole fruits and vegetables without doubling up from the pain that is sure to attack them after taking juices.

What is good advice for the colitis patient is good advice for everybody—*stick to whole fruits and vegetables,* rather than merely the juice. Canned, frozen or home-squeezed orange juice may be a very "convenient" way of introducing fruit into the breakfast menu, but it's most assuredly not a nutritionally correct way of introducing an orange into your digestive tract.

A final word on "home" digestive aids: *The kindest thing you can do for your stomach is not to overload it.*

Five or six smaller meals throughout the waking hours are far more sensible—and valuable to the preservation of your youthfulness—than three routine stuffings a day. I don't know who ever decreed that three times a day we must eat enough to assuage all hunger pangs throughout our sixteen, or more, waking hours. But whoever it was certainly had little practical knowledge of human physiology. The stomach that is overloaded once every five to six hours during the day is the stomach that gets "old" long before the rest of its body.

But the stomach that is given a smaller quantity of food (and I emphatically do not mean the junky between-meal piecing that is the rule rather than the exception in this country) every three to four hours is the stomach that will show its appreciation for this wise treatment by remaining healthy—and allowing its nearest neighbor, the *heart,* to avoid a lot of strain.

I was interested in reading an interview with the incomparable Mary Garden whose years are utterly belied by the youthfulness of her keen mind and lovely body.

"In all the years of my career," she told the reporter interviewing her, "I never ate those eight-and-ten-course dinners. I have never in my life overeaten! I like everything inside the animal. Liver, tongue, sweetbreads, I adore. And vegetables out of the garden. But out of the can, no. Bread I never touched—I was 'way ahead of my time."

In a few terse sentences, Mary Garden has summed up the essence of good nutrition—the essence of eating to *remain* young.

FOOD HABITS THAT PREVENT INSOMNIA

Insomnia has been treated at length in a previous book, *Health through Nutrition.* If you are a chronic victim of sleeplessness, then I recommend that you also read this more detailed treatment of the subject.

But for the purposes of your Eat-and-Grow-Younger program, I shall present here the nutritional side of preventing, or combating, insomnia—one of the most relentless foes of your efforts to stay young. And then, fortified with the food facts about sleep, you should make it a habit to eat for a good night's rest.

Before I tell you the foods that induce sleep, let me name two offenders that can bring on insomnia—too much starch, and too much common *table salt*. (I pass quickly over alcohol, coffee and tobacco as stimulants that can keep your nerves keyed up beyond the relaxing point. Enough has already been written about overindulgence in these powerful stimulants as a cause for insomnia.)

A highly revealing experiment on insomnia was conducted by Dr. Michael M. Miller, Associate Physician of St. Elizabeth's Hospital in Washington, D.C. His simple, *drugless* treatment consisted wholly of reducing the amount of table salt in the diet to the correct proportion. I have long been a crusader against the American habit of pouring excessive table salt into food, and it is encouraging to see that medical research, too, is beginning to recognize the insidious harm done to the human mechanism in a dozen different ways by too much of this far-from-harmless chemical.

Every food we eat already contains an adequate portion of natural salts from the earth. Under normal conditions, our bodies use less than 5 grams of salt a day. (Bear in mind that "salt" does not necessarily mean *sodium chloride* which is the chemical term for common table salt.) Yet most Americans consume between 10 and 30 grams of sodium chloride a day, in addition to the natural salts already present in the foods they eat.

The patients studied in Dr. Miller's experiment were allowed only 0.5 to 2 grams of table salt daily. All of the twenty patients were suffering from insomnia and nervous tension. One man was so tense he could not concentrate sufficiently to read, while three others suffered from severe headaches that contributed to their physical misery.

After no longer than a week on this low-salt diet, the patients began showing signs of the desirable physical tiredness which must take place at the end of the waking hours to balance mental tension before sleep can quiet the body. Within this comparatively short time of only *seven days,* these confirmed insomniacs were able to fall asleep within fifteen minutes or so after getting into bed. Better yet, most of them slept the night through without waking up. Those who did happen to wake up were able to go right back to sleep again within a few minutes, something any insomniac will recognize as a rare accomplishment. Some of the patients were even able to start taking regular afternoon naps—a wonderful youth-preservative for the past-forty body. After only a few more weeks on this low-salt diet, the patients reported either a marked decline in, or total absence of the disturbing dreams that had plagued them previous to the experiment.

In order to make certain that the effect of the treatment was more physical than psychological, after several weeks more salt was added to the diet of thirteen of the former insomniacs without their knowledge. Sure enough, it took only a week to ten days before they grew tense again, and began having difficulty sleeping.

Three of the twenty insomniacs did not respond satisfactorily to the low-salt diet, receiving no appreciable relief from their nervousness and inability to sleep. I would have liked to have tried an experiment of my own with those three persons. In addition to restricting the amount of table salt in their diets, I would have added liberal amounts of *calcium, lactic acid, vitamin C* and *vitamin-B-complex,* particularly *thiamine.*

So convinced am I that this combination of a low-salt diet with a diet rich in calcium, lactic acid, vitamin C and thiamine will restore the proper balance to the *chemistry of sleep* that I urge anyone troubled with stubborn insomnia, and the nerve tenseness that contributes to sleeplessness, to try for himself this safe dietary experiment.

We are not born into this world with the need to learn how to sleep as we must learn how to walk, talk or write. Sleep is as natural to the body as breathing, and a newborn baby does not have to be trained to sleep. It is only in later years as an adult, after he has allowed the habits of *unnatural* living to make deep inroads in his physical and mental health, that he must resort to artificial means for inducing the sleep that should be as instinctive with him as it is with the animal.

In your bloodstream should flow the only *sleep-inducers* needed by a healthy body to make possible the enjoyment of a good night's rest. The chemistry of the bloodstream has been so expertly worked out by nature that the blood flowing through your body is intended to be equipped for taking care of any bodily function, including that of sleep. It is only when this intricately balanced blood chemistry is upset that the body mechanism gets out of order, causing—among other things— insomnia.

The sleeping and waking of your body is controlled by a complex mechanism in the very depths of your brain, known as the *sleep center*. And this sleep center deep within your brain can be regulated in only one way—by your bloodstream. By a simple, ingenious method, nature has set up a *sleep cycle* between the brain, the nerves, the muscles, the bloodstream, then back to the brain again. This sleep cycle, when operating efficiently because the body chemistry is in balance, makes it utterly impossible for the conscious mind not to sleep at regular intervals whenever the body needs re-energizing.

This is the way the chemically controlled sleep cycle operates: Every time your brain sends out an action message to a muscle via a nerve of the central nervous system, certain chemical substances are secreted at the point of contact between the nerve and the muscles that are to go into action. One of the substances liberated at the nerve ends is *calcium*. During your waking hours, various muscles are continually being stimulated. This means that a lot of calcium is being liberated from the contact points between nerves and muscles. And all this calcium passes into the bloodstream, finally reaching the sleep center of your brain.

When enough calcium has been carried to the sleep center, automatically your conscious brain ceases to send out nerve impulses to your muscles. In other words, you have fallen asleep. And you fell asleep for the simple reason that the sleep center in your brain had become saturated with *calcium*.

In other words, the sleep center in your brain must be "sensitized" by special fatigue substances, such as *lactic acid,* before it can react to the influence of the *calcium* accumulations.

Therefore, your bloodstream must contain enough calcium plus enough lactic acid before the sleep center of your brain can produce the drowsiness and inactivity of your conscious mind that makes you "go to sleep."

If you are performing strenuous labor, or indulging in active outdoor exercise, the chances of your becoming an insomniac are slim. I've never met a laborer, a farmer, a lumberjack or a football player who suffered from insomnia. What's more, after a day spent in the outdoors, at the beach, or in the country, confirmed insomniacs of years' standing have been known to fall asleep as soon as their heads touched the pillow. Why? Partly because the sunshine and fresh air induced mental and physical relaxation, but principally because the greater amount of physical activity released more *calcium* and *lactic acid* into their bloodstream, thereby furnishing enough of these two body chemicals to "feed" the sleep center of the brain.

All the victims of sleeplessness whom I have observed are persons whose mental activity far overbalances their muscular activity. This means that not enough *calcium* and *lactic acid* are released into the bloodstream by hard-working muscles. The result is a sleep center that lacks sufficient of these two natural sleep-inducing chemicals to "knock out" the conscious brain long enough for the body to enjoy a period of complete relaxation.

And when to this systemic lack of calcium and lactic acid is added the further sin of meals also seriously deficient in mineral calcium and the lactic acid provided by soured milk, and sour-milk products, how can the average sedentary person living on an unbalanced diet expect to sleep as nature intended he should!

Balance the *sleep chemistry of your blood* and you can forget about counting sheep. You can then toss your sleeping pills into the garbage can where they belonged in the first place.

Because buttermilk, yogurt and cottage cheese made from soured milk are rich in both calcium and lactic acid, they are wonderful foods for persons who cannot produce enough of these two sleep-inducing chemicals through their own physical activity to feed the sleep center in the brain. That is why you will find many dishes using cottage cheese, soured powdered skim milk and buttermilk (yogurt, too) in the menus and recipes given in Part II.

And, to round out your diet-for-a-good-night's-rest, you must not overlook the B-vitamins, especially *thiamine*. Medical studies have disclosed that when you don't get enough thiamine (vitamin B-1) in your diet, you may become overly conscious of every twist and turn that it's normal for your sleeping body to make during the night to relieve the strain placed on certain muscles when your body lies prone. The slightest noise may awaken you, or the room may seem "too light." When these things happen to interrupt your sleep, your tense, unable-to-relax nerves are crying out for thiamine.

These are some of the foods rich in thiamine: Seed cereals, particularly sunflower seeds and millet, whole grains, eggs, chicken, fish roe, sardines, codfish, lean beef and mutton, liver, kidney, heart and brains. Try increasing the amount of these foods in your daily meals and decreasing the number of sweets and starches which overenergize your body to the point where it is "jumpy" during the day, and restless at night.

Indigestion (that includes constipation) is another well-known cause of broken sleep—another reason why high-starch meals for the person past-forty are likely to interrupt the natural sleep cycle. It's also true, as a rule, that if you indulge in rich, starchy meals you grossly neglect the natural foods that are good sources of the B-vitamins. So what these high-starch meals do is to clog up your digestive tract and starve your nerves at the same time—a perfect setup for insomnia.

A generous intake of *vitamin C,* another food element vital to your ability to get a good night's rest, helps prevent your blood vessels from losing *tone,* thereby impairing the circulation to the sleep center of your brain.

So let's have more emphasis on the body's chemical elements of sleep—*calcium, lactic acid, thiamine* and *vitamin C*—and less promoting of the extremely dangerous phenobarbital and bromide sleeping tablets by the drug industry. Sleep should be natural, not drugged.

These, then, are the principal bad habits that can help put the skids under your dream of enjoying a long "youth":

1. Too much starch, too little protein and a mineral-and-vitamin shortage
2. Stuffing yourself with large meals
3. Poor digestion
4. Restless, wakeful nights

Like a clever detective who ticks off, one by one, each clue that helps him solve a baffling crime, you should tick off each of these bad-habit menaces to your hopes of achieving a prolonged youthfulness.

When you have replaced these bad eating habits with the Six Commandments for a Long Youth (see Chapter 9), you will have started solving the crime that's being committed by none other than yourself against your chances for a long life, and a vigorous one, enjoyed in a body that stays *young-looking.*

Part II: YOUR EAT-AND-GROW-YOUNGER DIET PROGRAM

Chapter 22

START NOW TO EAT-AND-GROW-YOUNGER

PURPOSELY I have kept your diet program simple and easy to follow in order to make it flexible enough to fit anyone, under whatever personal condition or circumstance, in any place.

I could give you a detailed diet program, hour by hour and meal by meal, throughout the day. For example, I could specify that at 10:45 A.M. you were to drink a glass of this-and-that. But suppose you were not in a place or circumstance at that hour where such a drink were obtainable. You'd have to skip part of a consciously designed program.

And that would be extremely bad for the habit-forming psychology of your subconscious mind. Far better to have a flexible, readily adaptable Basic Menu, and then follow its *principles,* rather than to try following, item by item, a detailed diet program.

Therefore, I have made your Eat-and-Grow-Younger diet program so foolproof that it will be harder to skip or cheat than to follow it to the letter. Instead of a set of detailed menus, I have prepared adaptable diet schedules applicable to different conditions. That's why I have included a rather comprehensive set of recipes in the following chapters, so you may substitute one scheduled item for another (either another given recipe, or a similar one of your own preference, so long as it contains the same basic high-protein ingredients, or their equivalents).

High-protein dishes (those containing meats, fish, poultry, cheese, milk, sour cream, buttermilk, eggs, seed cereals and protein meat substitutes) may be interchanged from one day's menu to another without upsetting a calculated daily protein intake of approximately 150 to 165 grams.

After trying the Basic Menu for a while, if you find that this amount of daily protein does not quite meet your full energy requirements, you may increase your intake in whatever proportions you find effective for your highly individualized body needs.

An inexpensive, wholly effective, low-calorie way of obtaining increased protein (extra calcium, too) is by adding as much as 6 to 8 tablespoons of powdered skim milk to various dishes and beverages throughout the day.

Cottage cheese, too, provides another reasonably priced, high-protein (and calcium) food.

Sunflower seed kernels and meal, as well as millet and sesame seeds, are valuable sources of high proteins, minerals and vitamins, so extremely concentrated that the addition of 3 to 4 tablespoons of any of these seed cereals to the daily diet yields an effective increase in grams of high-grade protein, together with other essential nutrients.

In fact, most of the recipes given have already been fortified wherever possible with these less expensive, high-protein foods.

Honey, maple syrup, sorghum molasses, or raw sugar are the only sweeteners permitted in your Eat-and-Grow-Younger diet regimen. If you cheat and use white sugar, I won't know about it—you'll only be defrauding your own body. If you've never used honey instead of white sugar to sweeten your coffee or tea, you can't appreciate how much better these beverages can taste.

Keep a pot of pure honey on the table; in fact, replace the sugar bowl with the honey pot. Make every single item of food you buy and eat contribute something in the way of essential proteins, minerals and vitamins toward helping you look and feel younger.

If you are a vegetarian, you may obtain the full benefit of this high-protein diet by replacing the meat dishes with the protein meat-substitute recipes (or similar ones) given in Chapter 24. However, for the sake of your health, and your dreams of feeling and looking younger, I hope you're a vegetarian with no prejudices against eggs, low-fat milk and cheese, for I cannot advise eliminating these valuable protein foods along with meat.

Planned diet most certainly does not mean "monotonous" diet. You'll find the listed recipes and food combinations as -

titillating to your taste buds as they are beneficial to your hopes of erecting a barrier against premature old age.

In addition to the sheer pleasure of good food, there is another reason why my high-protein, low-starch menus and recipes stress seasonings and unusual combinations of familiar foods to surprise and delight your sense of taste.

When the artificially, prodigally flavored sugar-and-starch foods to which you may have become addicted are taken away from your mealtime routine, your debauched taste buds are likely to cry out in protest.

And that's when you will begin craving the rich desserts, breads, pasty macaroni and spaghetti dishes, sweet carbonated drinks and artificially colored and flavored candies which you've trained your pampered sense of taste to demand.

But if I can prove to you that high-prótein, low-starch meals can be made equally delicious and satisfyingly well-seasoned, with taste thrills you've never reveled in before, then your taste buds will send along to your brain the message: "How wonderfully new and different everything tastes! Why have we never had food like this before?"

So when I suggest such-and-such an herb, combination of herbs, special seasonings, or unusual combinations of good, simple foods, there's a very definite reason behind my suggestion. And you'll derive far more benefit from this high-protein regimen if you follow these directions as far as possible, rather than ignore them by going on preparing your dishes in the same old way.

Moreover, if food gives you a real taste thrill, you actually *eat less*, are better nourished and avoid the dangers of overeating. Science has proved that if you really enjoy your meals, your appetite is more likely to be kept within sensible bounds.

But when food is not tasty, your unsatisfied sense of taste drives you on to eat more than you should of highly flavored, starchy desserts and sweets in an effort to satisfy a nagging hunger. Such craving for more and more food after you've already eaten is really a *taste-hunger* rather than an actual emptiness of the stomach.

Remember, then, every meal should be as much of an adventure in taste as though you were sitting down before exotic dishes served in some far-away land. You'll find many foreign recipes given in the following pages—recipes handed down in my family, and recipes I've collected in my various travels.

If you've always seasoned with "salt, pepper and onions" as 99 per cent of the cook books so unimaginatively specify, then for the sake of the taste pleasures you're missing, learn to use herbs and herb-flavored salt, experiment with other seasonings besides the highly spiced condiments which "anesthetize" your taste buds with their fiery flavors.

For instance, why ruin the superb flavor of a wonderful broiled steak that should be a masterpiece of good food by dusting it liberally with black pepper, then dousing it with a flavor-deadening condiment sauce?

Instead, try rubbing a steak lightly with garlic-flavored oil before it goes into the broiler—the oil helps seal in the juices —salt to taste *after* it comes from the broiler, squeeze a few drops of lemon juice over both sides of the hot steak.

This, I should explain, is the jealousy guarded flavoring secret of the master chef in one of the most noted steak houses (cabañas, they are called) in Buenos Aires, the city of good food.

Good nutrition is not a matter of income. Rather, it's a matter of *selection.*

Proper foods actually cost less than many of those that are woefully lacking in nourishment. Many an expensively provisioned table is tragically poor in nutritional values because of poor selection and improper preparation.

Yet no mystery surrounds planned high-protein diets. The one basic dietary rule underlying all the menus and recipes herein provided for you is simply this:

Increase your daily protein intake to at least 150 to 165 grams (more if you've been ill, are planning a reducing diet or indulge in strenuous physical activities); limit the starches and sugars to natural carbohydrates found in vitamin-and-mineral-rich fruits, vegetables, honey, unrefined raw sugar or molasses, whole grains and seed cereals.

This is a diet regimen guaranteed to provide your body with the maximum of high proteins, minerals and vitamins obtainable from today's food items ordinarily grown on soils whose mineral richness is not always as great as it could be with more farsighted agricultural practices.

By adding a good multiple-vitamin mineral formula, you can eliminate any guesswork on minerals and vitamins, thus achieving the ideal diet for any person.

But more particularly for those persons who are firmly convinced that proper eating can be the "fairy godmother" that will transform them into the physical being they would like to be, and into the mental and spiritual force they have always envisioned themselves as becoming.

Don't delay in setting out to make your dreams of regained youthfulness come true. Put the Basic Menu of the high-protein Eat-and-Grow-Younger diet program into practice, starting with your very next meal.

And, as you begin noting the wondrously beneficial effects of this enlightened manner of planning and preparing meals, write to me. I'm always interested in the personal successes of my readers.

Your mind and your body can remain youthful many years past your so-called "prime," if only you don't help fasten the shackles of a premature old age on yourself every time you sit down at the table. Eat to grow younger!

FOODS CHARTED BY PROTEIN CONTENT

The following charts are prepared to give you a rule-of-thumb guide as to the adequacy or inadequacy of each day's meals from the standpoint of how many grams of protein are consumed.

First I shall list the *animal proteins*, that is, the high-grade or complete proteins; then the incomplete or *vegetable proteins*.

Your goal is to eat a minimum of at least 100 to 150 grams of protein each day, preferably 150 to 165 grams, distributed throughout your three meals and one or two between-meal snacks. And at least *50 to 75 per cent of your total daily protein consumption should be selected from the animal proteins*. The remainder of your daily protein intake may come from vegetable sources.

Immediately following these charts is shown a Basic High-Protein Menu, together with a sample menu as a guide to apportioning your quota of protein grams.

ANIMAL PROTEINS

Quantity	Food	Protein Grams
1 cup	beef broth	4
1 slice (4 oz.)	lean beef (rib, rump, pot roast)	22
1 serving (4 oz.)	beefsteak	23
1 serving (4 oz.)	corned beef, canned or fresh	16
1 serving (4 oz.)	beef tongue	16
1 serving (4 oz.)	beef sweetbreads	14
1 serving (4 oz.)	beef heart	17
1 serving (4 oz.)	beef liver	20
1 slice (4 oz.)	lamb, roast	22
2 average	lamb chops	20
1 serving (4 oz.)	lamb's liver	20
1 slice (4 oz.)	mutton, roast leg	20

ANIMAL PROTEINS—Continued

Quantity	Food	Protein Grams
1 serving (4 oz.)	veal cutlets	20
2 (4 oz.)	veal chops	19
1 serving (4 oz.)	veal, roast leg	23
1 serving (4 oz.)	calves' liver	23
1 serving (4 oz.)	chicken	18
½ cup	chicken livers	20
1 serving (4 oz.)	duck	21
1 serving (4 oz.)	goose	22
1 serving (4 oz.)	turkey	24
6 (¾ cup)	clams	14
1 serving (4 oz.)	codfish	16
⅔ cup	crabmeat	16
1 serving (4 oz.)	pan fish, average fresh-water	21
1 serving (4 oz.)	herring	19
½ cup	lobster meat, canned	16
7 medium	oysters	6
4 average	sardines, canned	13
6 filets	anchovies	10
½ cup (4 oz.)	salmon, canned	22
4 oz.	scallops	16
6 medium	shrimp	8
¼ cup (4 oz.)	tuna, canned	9
1 serving (4 oz.)	whitefish	22
1 serving (4 oz.)	rabbit	20
1 whole	egg	6
1 whole	egg white	3
1 whole	egg yolk	3
½ cup	egg custard, fortified with 4 extra tbsp. powdered skim milk	15 to 18
1 cube (2x1x1 in.)	American cheese	12
2 tbsp.	Cheddar cheese	7
2 tbsp.	Italian cheese, grated	12
½ cup	cottage cheese	20
1 tbsp.	cream cheese	2
1 slice	Swiss cheese	10
1 qt.	buttermilk	30
1 qt.	yogurt	30
1 qt.	fresh whole milk	33
1 qt.	fresh skim milk	34
½ cup	powdered skim milk	53
5 tbsp.	powdered skim milk	34
½ cup	evaporated (canned) milk	8

ANIMAL PROTEINS—Continued

Quantity	Food	Protein Grams
4 tbsp.	table cream, 20%	2
4 tbsp.	whipping cream, 40%	1
1 serving (1 cup)	cream vegetable soup, made with fortified milk, with sunflower or sesame meal added	12
1 serving (1 cup)	cream soup, containing eggs or cheese and made as above	20 to 24
½ cup	ice cream, homemade, made with eggs and fortified milk	8 to 10
½ cup	ice cream, commercial	2
1 tbsp.	gelatin powder, unflavored	8
1 tbsp.	honey (an animal protein)	2
	sunflower seeds	38% to 52%*
	millet meal	11% to 23%*
	sesame seeds	19% to 32%*
2 tbsp.	peanuts	23% to 30%*
	almonds	20% to 28%*

The next chart lists the vegetable sources providing the highest number of protein grams per serving. By this I do not intend to imply that no other vegetable sources are worth considering. It's merely that space does not permit listing them all, so I have been forced to select those sources which will yield the most protein with the least bulk, and with the greatest degree of digestibility.

Since these vegetable proteins are not high-grade, or "complete," no more than 25 per cent, or approximately one fourth, of your daily protein intake should be chosen from this list:

VEGETABLE PROTEINS

Quantity	Food	Protein Grams
8 halves	apricots, dried	1
6 halves	apricots, fresh	1
1 medium	artichoke, Jerusalem	1
8 stalks	asparagus, green	2
½ medium	avocado	2
1 medium	banana (black-ripe)	1
½ cup	kidney beans	6

* Not animal proteins, but high-grade.

VEGETABLE PROTEINS—Continued

Quantity	Food	Protein Grams
½ cup	lima beans, dry	8
½ cup	lima beans, green	7
¾ cup	green string beans	2
½ cup	beets	2
1 slice	rye bread (whole-grain)	3
1 slice	whole-grain bread, fortified with milk powder, and millet meal, sunflower seed or sesame seed meal	5
¾ cup	broccoli (leaf, stem and flower)	3
¾ cup	brussels sprouts	4
5 tbsp.	buckwheat, whole	12
1 cup	cabbage, raw (green or Chinese)	2
½ cup	carrots, sliced or diced	1
¾ cup	cauliflower	2
4 stalks	celery, green	1
½ cup	celery root	3
½ cup	chard leaves, cooked	2
12 large	cherries	1
3 tbsp.	coconut	1
½ cup	collard greens, cooked	3
½ cup	corn, yellow, canned	4
1 medium	corn, yellow on cob	3
½ cup	cornmeal, unbolted	8
1 medium	cucumber	1
½ cup	dandelion greens, cooked	3
15 medium	dates	3
½ cup	eggplant	1
10 stalks	endive	1
¾ cup	escarole (chicory)	1
2 small	figs, dried	1
2 large	figs, fresh	1
1 cup	buckwheat flour	6
1 cup	whole-wheat flour	12
¾ cup	gooseberries	1
1 small bunch	grapes	1
1 average	guava	1
½ cup	huckleberries	1
½ cup	kale, cooked	4
½ cup	kohlrabi, cooked	2
½ cup	leeks	2
½ cup	lamb's-quarters (greens)	4
½ cup	lentils	9

VEGETABLE PROTEINS—Continued

Quantity	Food	Protein Grams
10 leaves	lettuce, green	1
¼ head	lettuce, bleached	1
1 cup	loganberries, canned	1
⅓ small	cantaloupe	1
1 medium	muffin, whole-grain with millet, sunflower or sesame meal	2
¾ cup	mushrooms	4
½ cup	mustard greens, cooked	2
½ cup	oatmeal, steel-cut	4
½ cup	okra	2
2 small, dry	onions	1
½ cup	parsley	6
½ cup	parsnips	2
3 halves	peaches, dried	1
2 large halves	peaches, canned or fresh	1
½ cup	peas, dried	12
½ cup	fresh green peas	7
10 large	pecans	3
1 medium	green pepper	1
1 large	persimmon	2
2 medium	red pimento	1
3 medium	plums	1
1 medium	white potato, baked or boiled in jacket	3
1 medium	sweet potato, baked	3
6 medium	prunes, dried	2
½ cup	pumpkin, cooked	1
15 large	radishes	1
¼ cup	raisins	1
½ cup	raspberries	1
¾ cup	brown rice, cooked	4
¾ cup	rutabagas	1
2 roots	salsify (oyster plant)	3
½ cup	squash, Hubbard or summer, cooked	1
½ cup	strawberries	1
2 medium	tangerines	1
1 large	orange	1
1 medium	grapefruit	1
½ cup	tomatoes, canned	1
1 medium	tomato, fresh	1
½ cup	tomato juice, canned	2
½ cup	turnips, cooked	1

VEGETABLE PROTEINS—Continued

Quantity	Food	Protein Grams
½ cup	turnip greens	2
¼ cup	walnuts, English	5
½ cup	wheat germ, raw	24

BASIC HIGH-PROTEIN MENU IF YOUR WEIGHT IS NORMAL

Breakfast

Fresh or cooked fruit
Choice of two:

1 serving of eggs (2 eggs), fish, meat (no bacon or ham)
1 serving whole-grain toast, *if you must*—spread with cheese instead of butter
1 serving millet mush or porridge
1 serving cheese (cube of American cheese, or ½ cup cottage cheese, either served plain, or mixed with fresh fruit; or in an omelet or pancakes)
2 tbsp. powdered skim milk, liquefied and used as beverage, or incorporated into the egg or porridge
Beverage, sweetened with honey if desired

Mid-Morning Snack (optional)

Milk drink (buttermilk, yogurt or milk shake), fresh or dried fruit

Lunch

1 cup clear soup or broth
1 serving meat, fish, poultry, eggs, cheese (alternate this selection with whatever choice was made for the main breakfast dish, i.e., if eggs are chosen for breakfast, select meat, fish, poultry or cheese for lunch)
1 serving raw green vegetables, either in bowl or finger salad
1 serving of protein dessert, such as custard, gelatin, fruit pudding, etc.
Beverage, if desired

Mid-Afternoon Snack (optional)

Milk drink (buttermilk, yogurt, fortified milk shake or herb tea)

Dinner

1 cup light broth (beef or chicken)
1 serving meat, fish, poultry, meat substitutes, cheese, or eggs (again the selection alternates with the high-protein entrees chosen for previous meals)
1 serving cooked vegetable
1 serving tossed or finger salad
1 serving fruit dessert
Beverage, if desired

If fortified with such highly concentrated complete-protein foods as powdered skim milk, sunflower seeds (and meal), millet and sesame seeds (and meal) wherever possible, this Basic Menu should yield a total daily protein consumption of anywhere from 165 to 200 grams.

Here is one day's sample menu worked out from the Basic Menu, using the recipes given in the chapters that follow:

SAMPLE HIGH-PROTEIN MENU FOR NORMAL WEIGHT

Breakfast

1 dish sliced oranges, plain or served with fresh or canned berries
1 small bowl of Millet Porridge cooked in half water and half non-fat fortified milk
1 serving Cottage Cheese Omelet
Beverage, sweetened with honey if desired

Lunch

1 cup clear Soup or broth
1 slice cold roast beef, lamb or poultry
Finger salad (celery, pepper, carrot, cucumber, etc. strips and slices)
1 serving (½ cup) Lemon Milk Sherbet
Beverage, sweetened with honey if desired

Dinner

1 cup beef or chicken broth

1 serving Meat Cakes
1 serving Gourmet's Salad
1 serving (½ cup) Fruit Custard
Beverage, sweetened with honey if desired

By interchanging the recipes given in this sample menu with the others of similar value in the corresponding chapters, or with those of your own preference (always provided they are made with the same high-protein, whole-grain, no-white-sugar ingredients), you can work out an endless succession of menus far better adapted to your individual needs and circumstances than if I were to work out a set of menus for you.

If your bathroom scales insinuate that you need to lose weight, then by all means do so. But first make certain that you're really overweight. Reducing for the sake of sheer vanity is risky business. Don't take chances with your health by losing weight you can't afford to shed.

Yet if you, your scales and the family doctor all agree that your health (and good looks, too) would benefit by getting rid of a few pounds, then the one and only *safe* reducing diet is that built around plenty of high-protein foods, mainly meats.

Of course, such a reducing diet is going to cost you money —but so does ill health, and obesity is synonymous with ill health and early loss of your youth. So look upon the money spent on this high-protein diet as an *investment in health*.

The following High-Protein Reducing Menu is designed to produce a weight loss of no more than 5 to 8 pounds a month. To lose more quickly than this is dangerous. Of course, your weight may hold steady for a week or two at a time, then drop down 5 pounds or more all at once; or you may lose a lot right at the start, then not lose any more for several weeks. But the over-all loss should not exceed 5 to 8 pounds a month, that is, if you value your appearance and wish to avoid the haggard look so commonly associated with dieting.

If you find that you lose more than 5 to 8 pounds on the following Basic High-Protein Reducing Menu, then increase your portions. If, on the other hand, you find you don't lose more than 3 to 4 pounds a month, you may omit the bread. But, of course, this brings up the danger of a B-vitamin deficiency. So under such circumstances, you should be content with a 3 to 4 pound steady weight loss and not run the risk of incurring a serious vitamin or mineral deficiency.

You may vary or adapt this Basic High-Protein Reducing

Menu as you wish, interchanging one high-protein meat, fish or fowl with another; and alternating eggs with cheese. But you should confine the major portion of your fruit and vegetable consumption to those listed as *5 per cent* and *10 per cent carbohydrates* in the chart which follows the menu.

BASIC HIGH-PROTEIN REDUCING DIET

Breakfast

- 1 small orange, or half grapefruit, unsweetened
- 1 slice cold meat, fish, or chicken; or 1 pan-broiled minute steak
- 1 boiled, poached or shirred egg (also scrambled over hot water); *or* 1-inch cube of cheese, or ¼ cup of cottage cheese

Small bowl of Millet Porridge eaten with non-fat milk
- 1 cup hot skim milk sweetened with ¼ teaspoon of honey; or black coffee or tea, sweetened with a little honey if desired

Mid-Morning

- 1 small glass skim milk, buttermilk or yogurt; or tomato juice fortified by whipping in a little cottage cheese

Lunch

- 1 cup clear, skimmed broth
- 1 slice broiled or roasted meat, fish, poultry (don't overlook liver in this diet)
- 1 green salad, dressed either with lemon juice and very little salt, or with ¼ cup of cottage cheese seasoned with minced chives
- 1 serving of fresh 5% or 10% fruit

Hot beverage, sweetened with honey only

Mid-Afternoon

- 1 small glass of skim milk, either hot or cold and flavored with a little crushed fresh or cooked fruit

Dinner

- 1 cup beef or skimmed chicken broth
- 1 serving meat, fish or poultry

1 serving cooked green vegetable such as asparagus or
   broccoli, served with plain lemon juice; or a tossed green
   salad similar to the one eaten at lunch
1 slice whole-grain bread (only if you *must*)
1 serving egg custard, or milk sherbet made with skim milk
   or buttermilk, and fortified with extra powdered skim milk

This is far from being a "starvation" menu, and I promise
you won't have a lank, gnawing feeling in the pit of your
stomach while following this reducing diet. Nor will you
suffer any loss of energy. On the contrary, you'll feel like a
new person as soon as all that high-protein food begins to
take hold, and as the unnecessary poundage melts away.

Another wise precaution is to fortify yourself against possible deficiencies by taking a good multiple vitamin mineral
concentrate. Dietary supplements are always good sense in
any reducing regimen (but make certain you buy a reliable
product).

Now here are the more common fruits and vegetables
classified as to their carbohydrate content, that is, to the pro-
portionate number of calories they contain:

5% VEGETABLES AND FRUITS (Low-Starch)

VEGETABLES

Asparagus	Lettuce
Bean Sprouts	Mushrooms
Brussels sprouts	Okra
Cabbage	Olives
Cauliflower	Peppers
Celery	Pumpkin
Cucumbers	Radishes
Eggplant	String beans
Endive	Summer Squash
Greens	Swiss Chard
Kohlrabi	Tomatoes
Leeks	Watercress

FRUITS

Cantaloupe	Lemons
Honeydew Melon	Watermelon

10% VEGETABLES AND FRUITS (Low-Starch)

VEGETABLES

Beets
Carrots
Onions
Oyster plant (salsify)

Rutabagas
Squash (Hubbard, acorn,
   baking, etc.)
Turnips

FRUITS

Blackberries
Cranberries
Currants
Gooseberries

Grapefruit
Limes
Oranges
Peaches
Strawberries

15% VEGETABLES AND FRUITS
VEGETABLES

Lima beans, green
Parsnips

Peas, green

FRUITS

Apples
Apricots
Blueberries
Cherries, sour
Grapes
Loganberries

Mulberries
Pears
Pineapple
Plums
Raspberries

20% FRUITS AND VEGETABLES

VEGETABLES

Beans (dried or canned):
   lima
   kidney
   navy
Corn
Potatoes

FRUITS

Bananas
Cherries, sweet
Grape juice

ABOUT THE RECIPES THAT FOLLOW

Each recipe is usually enough to serve four persons, and
I have tried to indicate where a greater number of servings

is prepared. By means of simple arithmetic, it's easy enough to prepare these same recipes for one or two. Even when a recipe calls for one egg, no insurmountable problem is faced. Merely break and beat the egg as directed in the recipe. Then with a measuring spoon use what would be approximately one-half or one-fourth of the total egg, saving the remainder in a tightly covered dish in the refrigerator for use in another halved or quartered one-egg recipe. However, if you don't have any serious aversion to leftovers, prepare the whole recipe and refrigerate or deep-freeze what is left, thereby enjoying that much extra time saved from meal preparation on another day.

In recipes where hard-cooked eggs are used, to save time the eggs may be boiled the night before (earlier in the day, also), put in the refrigerator and peeled immediately before using. Also, a day's supply of liquefied powdered skim milk may be made up the night before and kept in the refrigerator in a tightly covered bottle or jar. The thickened milk sauce called for in many cheese and egg dishes may also be prepared the night before, then refrigerated and reheated before using. I mention these time-saving breakfast-recipe tips in the hope that, with more efficiency, breakfast will cease to be the slapdash meal into which it has now degenerated.

You'll notice that many of the recipes in all chapters call for yogurt, sour milk or buttermilk. If none of these are on hand, it's easy enough to make sour milk or buttermilk by adding two tablespoons of lemon juice to one cup of sweet milk. Instead of lemon juice, a good grade of wine- or honey-vinegar does just as well.

And don't skip the delicious yogurt recipes because you don't have, or can't get, yogurt. One cup of yogurt may be effectively replaced in a recipe by one cup of sour milk or buttermilk (and you've already learned how to achieve this with sweet milk and lemon juice or vinegar). So if you have milk, either fresh or powdered, on your pantry shelf, and lemons in the fruit bag, you are all set to try any of the recipes calling for buttermilk, sour milk or yogurt. Cooking with yogurt, buttermilk and sour milk is one way of adding extra protein (lactic acid, too) to your diet without spending a lot of money.

Also, steaks, or the tougher cuts of meat, if marinated overnight in sour milk or buttermilk, are made much more tender and flavorful. And by changing the buttermilk every couple of days, the steak may be kept for a week, acquiring greater tenderness and flavor the longer it marinates in the lactic acid. I am told this is an old camping trick—to immerse fresh meat in sour milk or buttermilk in order to preserve it where no refrigeration is possible. A flank steak, ordinarily a very tough cut, allowed to soak for several days in buttermilk and then swissed, is deliciously tender. But I'm getting ahead of my story on meats!

Throughout this book, and in the recipes that follow, you'll find these and other foods mentioned:

millet	whole grains
sunflower seeds	natural flours
sesame seeds	dried fruits
kelp	molasses, unbleached
sea salt	skim milk powder
raw sugar	vitamin-mineral food
pure honey	supplements
safflower and	yogurt
other oils	lecithin granules
brown rice	wheat germ

With the exception of powdered skim milk, brown rice and molasses—you'll find it next to impossible to purchase unprocessed, 100% natural foods in the regular markets.

You must, therefore, turn to your nearest health food store as a source of these, and other nutritious products: A check in the pages of your telephone directory can help you locate such a store.

Originally established to provide only natural foods, the health food store grew rapidly into an important source of specialized foods that you cannot find elsewhere.

If you live in an area not served by a health food store, you can order by mail from one nearest you. And, after locating a health food store, you find it does not carry a particular food you want—ask them to order it for you. A little effort and patience on your part will give you the kind of health-maintaining foods you want and should have.

SOME GENERAL HINTS

Here are a few general hints regarding the ingredients used in recipes that follow. These hints may well serve as guides to all of your cooking:

where recipes call for:
SUGAR . . . use unrefined *raw sugar* instead of the ordinary white sugar which adds nothing to good nutrition.

SALT . . . in place of ordinary salt, use the variety known as *sea salt*. This provides additional natural minerals which ordinary salt does not.

OILS, cooking or salad . . . your first choice should be *safflower oil*, which provides many nutrition extras, being the oil richest in polyunsaturates. Other oils, in order of nutritional values: sunflower, sesame, rice bran, soybean, corn.

MOLASSES . . . do not used bleached or sulphured varieties. Get the kind known as blackstrap, sorghum or barbadoes.

MILK . . . for the most part, it is best to use fresh skim milk—(sold as non-fat milk in some areas)—or you can make "reconstituted" milk with skim milk powder. It is also a good idea to add some skim milk powder to fresh milk as a means of fortifying its protein and other values.

Now for the recipes.

Chapter 23

HIGH-PROTEIN MEATS, POULTRY AND FISH

LET me emphasize that you don't need to buy the most expensive cuts of meat in order to obtain the most protein nutrition from flesh foods. The cheaper cuts of beef and lamb, as well as their gland and organ meats, contain just as much, often more, nutrition as the most costly steaks, chops and roasts.

In addition, the proteins in fish and poultry are as valuable to your body as those to be had from beef or lamb. So don't bankrupt the budget in an effort to obtain the finest cut of meat in the butcher shop with the thought that it will be "better nutrition." It's not necessary. Get acquainted with the cheaper cuts, and above all try to cultivate—if you don't have already—a taste for highly nutritious liver, heart and brains.

I have tried to include recipes for as many types of flesh foods as might please the appetites of the average family, with greater emphasis on the less expensive meats so that you will have meat often—at least once, if not twice, a day if your budget permits. Otherwise no less frequently than every second day, with fill-ins of cheese, eggs and meat-substitute dishes on the days when meat, fish or poultry does not grace your table.

Remember always to cook all meats (other high-protein foods as well) slowly at low temperatures to conserve the proteins and vitamins, to avoid undue shrinkage, to obtain tenderer, juicier meat, and to avoid scorched drippings.

HIGH-PROTEIN MEAT LOAF

1 lb. ground meat (this may be all beef or lamb, all liver or heart, or a mixture of muscle and organ meats)
4 tbsp. wheat germ, or millet meal
4 tbsp. sunflower seed meal
1/3 cup powdered skim milk
1 egg, slightly beaten
2 tsp. lemon juice
1/4 cup non-fat milk

1 clove garlic
4 tbsp. finely chopped green pepper or red pimento
1 tbsp. cooking oil
1 tsp. salt
1/4 tsp. thyme
pinch of sweet basil
dash of nutmeg or mace
2 tbsp. grated Italian cheese, if desired

Let the peeled, split garlic clove soak in the liquid milk for at least 30 minutes to 1 hour before using. Mix all the ingredients in a large bowl, governing the amount of liquid milk according to the consistency—not too soft, nor yet too stiff to mold well. Shape into a large loaf and place in the greased bottom of a covered baking pan or small roaster. Spoon about 1/4 cup of tomato juice or diluted tomato paste over the top of the loaf. Cover and allow to bake in a moderate oven (350° F.) for 45 to 55 minutes, removing the cover for the last 10 minutes to allow slight browning on top. This is your basic meat-loaf recipe, to be used as presented, or adapted in any variations that occur to you, or that fit the ingredients you have on hand. You'll find this high-protein meat loaf as delicious cold as hot, and it makes a splendid low-cost meat for lunch boxes or buffet suppers. If you want to garnish it, arrange crescents of hard-cooked egg with strips of red pimento and hulled sunflower seeds into flower and petal designs on top of the loaf after it comes from the oven. By serving this high-protein entrée at least once a week, allowing for some to be left over for lunches or a meal the next day, you will find the meat budget stretching further than you had expected.

SAVORY POT ROAST

3 to 4 lbs. pot roast (chuck, rump, shoulder or heel of round)
3 tbsp. cooking oil

1 clove garlic
2 tbsp. grated lemon rind
2 cups yogurt
salt to taste

Rub the roast well with salt and the cut halves of the garlic clove. Then place the garlic in the yogurt to flavor it. Rub the entire roast with about ⅓ of the cooking oil in order to seal in the juices and flavor. Heat the remainder of the oil in a Dutch oven or heavy, deep, iron skillet which can be tightly covered. Brown the roast lightly in the oil, add the grated lemon rind, allowing to simmer a few minutes before pouring the yogurt over the roast and spooning up the pan gravy with the lemon rind over the meat to let the flavor penetrate into the roast. Cover and cook over a very slow fire for about 2½ to 3 hours, basting the meat often to avoid drying and sticking to the pan. About 30 minutes before the meat is done (and remember that the yogurt will help tenderize it), add 3 or 4 cleaned whole carrots to brown in the sauce around the meat. This produces the most tasty pot roast you've ever eaten. The garlic clove may be left in the sauce for the first 30 minutes, then removed. This roast is excellent for slicing cold, and it's one leftover the family won't mind seeing the second day in a row. When served cold, add to the menu a hot baked potato, a cooked green vegetable and a fruit mold.

HUNGARIAN LAMB

3 lbs. shoulder lamb cut into small cubes
1 cup yogurt
2 cups tomato juice, or 4 tbsp. tomato paste diluted with 3 cups water
2 small onions

2 tbsp. cooking oil (or butter)
1 tbsp. minced parsley
½ tsp. salt
dash of paprika
sprig of fresh sweet marjoram, or a pinch each of dried marjoram and summer savory

Heat the oil in a Dutch oven or covered chicken fryer, add the finely minced onions and brown lightly. Add the cubes of lamb from which all fat and tendons have been removed, and into which the salt and paprika have been well rubbed. Allow to brown lightly. Stir in the tomato juice, parsley and herbs. Cover and let simmer over a very low flame on top of the stove for about 2 hours. The covered skillet or Dutch oven may also be placed in a slow (300° to 325° F.) oven for about the same length of time. Add a little hot water if the sauce around the meat cooks low. Immediately before serving, stir in the yogurt, mixing it well with the meat and tomato juice. Garnish the platter with sprigs of fresh mint, if available. Even people who "don't like" lamb come back for a second helping of this delicious entrée.

BEEF CASSEROLE

1 lb. chuck beef	2 tbsp. cooking oil
2 tbsp. millet meal	1 cup stewed or canned tomatoes
1 tsp. salt	
¼ tsp. paprika	1 garlic clove
dash of mace or nutmeg	hot water

Cut the beef into one-inch cubes, roll in the millet meal into which have been blended the salt, paprika and nutmeg or mace. Heat the oil in a heavy skillet and brown the cubes lightly. Pour over them the tomatoes in which the clove of garlic has been soaking, removing the garlic if only a mild flavor is desired, otherwise allowing it to remain. Add enough hot water to cover. Bake in a covered casserole in a moderate over (350° F.) for about 2 hours, or until the meat cubes are tender. This is your "economy" dish, one that will provide a full quota of high protein for one meal's entree when your budget is running low.

CAMPFIRE BROILED STEAK (AT HOME!)

Nowhere does a steak taste as delicious as when broiled over an open fire. Of course open fires are out of the question in a modern kitchen, but you can broil your steak by the same principles that make the campfire steak "out of this world." Here's what you do: Rub your steak well with a cut clove of garlic, but *do not salt*. Place on the cold broiler rack, in an oven that has *not* been preheated, about 3 to 3½ inches below a very low flame—about as low as the flame can be without going out. Now, the whole secret hinges on leaving the broiler door open, so that the steak does not become dry from the too-great heat of the closed-in broiler. The secret of open-air cooking is that subtle mixture of hot and cool air which cooks the meat at the same time that it allows the steak to retain its natural juiciness. A steak cooked under this very low flame, with the broiler door open, will take longer, but it's worth every extra minute you wait for it! In order to even the browning, turn the steak several times, taking particular care not to pierce the meat with your fork, otherwise much valuable nutrition is lost in the juice that runs out. Try to put the fork in the fat, or hook it under the bone. Then when the steak is done to your taste, remove to a heated platter, salt both sides, squeeze a few drops of lemon juice over it, and allow a piece of butter to melt and blend into the juicy meat. Once you've broiled a steak this way, you'll never again waste another piece of expensive meat by ruining it in the old cooked-to-death, hurry-up, smell-up-the-house way. There is little or no splattering of grease in this low-fire, slow-cooking method of steak broiling, nor will the steak smell while cooking. Which, of course, means that you *eat* the food value that formerly was wasted by cooking temperatures so high that the delicious food smell reached your nostrils instead of your tummy.

Variation: Instead of salting the steak when it leaves the broiler, remove from the broiling pan a few minutes before the meat is done to your taste, spread the top side with softened Roquefort cheese, return to the broiler for a few minutes longer, then remove to a heated platter and garnish with chopped chives. This method of preparing a steak gives you a "double dose" of protein and is a real energy meal.

BROILED LIVER SUPREME

1 to 1½ lbs. calves' liver
1 garlic clove
3 tbsp. melted butter or cooking oil
½ tsp. salt
dash of mace or nutmeg
1 large onion cut in rings (optional)
1 scant tbsp. cooking wine or lemon juice

Prepare the liver by wiping with a damp cloth, and removing all skin and veins. Cut into slices about ½-inch thick for individual servings, and rub each side with the cut halves of the garlic clove. Sprinkle lightly with salt on both sides, dash the tiniest bit of mace or nutmeg on one side only, and brush both sides with melted butter or cooking oil. Place on a greased wire broiler about 2½ to 3 inches from a medium flame. If onion rings are used, place one on each slice after it has been brushed with the melted butter or cooking oil. Broil for about 5 minutes, then turn (first removing the onion rings to be replaced on the uncooked side). Continue broiling for another 5 minutes, or until done. Just before removing from the broiler, sprinkle a few drops of cooking wine or lemon juice on each piece of the broiled liver. The careful seasoning of the liver makes this one undisguised way to serve liver so that its taste appeals even to those who have a serious prejudice against eating this wonderful organ meat. Moreover, the slow, careful broiling and the sealing in of the juices by the melted butter or oil assures liver containing a maximum of its protein and vitamins.

BREADED BRAINS ITALIAN STYLE

2 lbs. calves' brains	1 cup millet meal
4 tbsp. cooking oil	1 tbsp. chopped parsley
1 tbsp. grated Italian cheese	salt to taste
(Romano or Parmesan)	

Wash the brains well, then cover with cold water to which about 1 tablespoon of lemon juice or wine vinegar and salt are added, and parboil for 5 minutes. Peel off all the outer membrane after removing from the water. Cut into portions of serving size. Roll in the millet meal into which has been blended the grated cheese, salt and chopped parsley. Heat the cooking oil in a skillet, and sauté the breaded portions for about 5 minutes, or until golden brown on both sides. This meat should be served immediately, squeezing a few drops of lemon juice over each portion (as you would with fish) before eating. Serve with a salad bowl, and a sliced fruit dessert. Brains served in this manner are a great delicacy in many Italian homes. It is one way of utilizing this cheaper organ meat so that, in my opinion, it is as delicious as the more expensive sweetbreads. Brains are one of the richest sources of the B-vitamin, *choline*.

FRIZZLED DRIED BEEF

Without tearing the paper-thin slices any more than can be helped, allow about ¼ cup per portion, and drop into a heated skillet containing hot melted butter. Allow to just heat through, which won't take more than several minutes if the butter is hot, since the slices are so thin. Dried beef contains lots of nourishment, and is usually an economical meat. Prepared in this manner, it makes a delicious breakfast meat to replace the accustomed bacon or ham as an accompaniment for eggs.

CHICKEN BAKED IN YOGURT

Disjoint a fresh stewing chicken, or use a packaged frozen chicken already disjointed, rubbing each piece well with salt.

Roll in millet meal as for fried chicken, put in a skillet with a small amount of heated cooking oil and brown each piece lightly on both sides. Remove from the skillet and arrange the pieces in a baking dish or deep casserole. Sprinkle lightly with sweet basil and chopped chives. Cover the chicken with 1 cup or so of yogurt. Cover tightly and allow to steam-bake in a slow oven (275° to 300° F.) for about 2 hours, or until tender. It's not necessary to buy the younger, more expensive chickens for this dish, since the yogurt and the low cooking heat will make a stewing chicken very tender. This is also a doubly nutritious way to serve chicken because of the extra protein and calcium obtained from the yogurt.

CHICKEN FROM TAHITI

1 large frying chicken, or 2 small ones (serves 4)
2 tbsp. cooking oil or butter (half oil and half butter is better than all butter because it lessens the tendency for the chicken to burn and stick)
½ tsp. salt
1 clove garlic

Sauce:

½ cup fresh or canned crushed pineapple
1 cup chopped Chinese cabbage (optional)
2 tbsp. chopped chives or leeks
2 medium stalks of celery, diced
½ cup shredded or chopped blanched almonds, or freshly grated coconut
½ cup chopped green peppers
1 small fresh tomato peeled and chopped, or 4 tbsp. drained canned tomato juice
2 tbsp. lemon juice or cooking wine

Cut the dressed chickens into pieces for frying, salt and sauté in the cooking oil in which the peeled clove of garlic has been allowed to heat. Use a covered chicken fryer, or a heavy iron skillet that may be covered. After the chicken is a nice golden brown on one side, turn, cover tightly, lower the flame and allow to cook very slowly until tender. It may be necessary to turn the pieces several times to prevent their sticking and burning. When done, place on a deep platter in the oven to keep warm while the sauce is being prepared. Place the chopped tomato, pepper, celery, Chinese cabbage and chives or leeks into the hot oil remaining in the skillet, season to taste with salt, cover and allow to steam until the celery and pepper are slightly softened, then add the pineapple and lemon juice or cooking wine. Heat through and remove from the fire. Pour this sauce over the chicken which has been kept warm meanwhile, and sprinkle with the almonds or grated fresh coconut. (Chopped sunflower seed kernels may be used instead with equally delicious results.) This makes another one-dish meal. Add a baked potato and a milk sherbet served with sesame seed cookies for a "party" meal that's both unusual and unusually nutritious.

ROAST FOWL WITH ORIENTAL STUFFING

This recipe has a very interesting story behind it, and I think you should hear it. I attended a dinner party one time in Bangkok, Siam, at which a parsimonious Chinese cook sent one lone duck to the table. The expression of my host as he carved and carved—in vain—is still very vivid. However, the flavor of ducks prepared by Chinese cooks, regardless of their devious methods of stretching the "market money," is most superior. The Chinese know more about fowl than any other people.

The stuffing was truly heavenly and, while native cooks do not like to divulge their culinary secrets, I managed with some persuasion to get this recipe. The cheese called for was obtainable only in Siam, but I found, by experimentation, that Romano was a perfect substitute.

May I suggest that the next time you have duck (or chicken or turkey) you try this truly excellent rice stuffing. I am sure you will vote it most pleasing. For a five or six pound bird, the following ingredients will suffice:

Stuffing:

1 cup brown rice
¼ cup cooking oil or melted butter
1 cup minced onion or chives (the latter give a milder flavor)
1 cup chopped celery and parsley
1 cup chopped green pepper
1 tsp. chopped garlic
1 large apple, peeled and diced
2 tbsp. grated Romano cheese
2 cups broth from cooked giblets
chopped giblets
¾ tsp. salt
3 tbsp. sunflower seed meal (optional)
pinch of thyme
pinch of sweet marjoram, leaf or powdered
dash of mace or nutmeg

2 eggs, beaten

pinch of summer savory
pinch of rosemary

Wash the brown rice. Use a deep heavy skillet and brown the rice lightly in half the melted shortening over a moderate fire. Add the broth from the cooked giblets, cover lightly and allow to cook over a slow fire for about 20 minutes, or until the rice is about half done. Meanwhile sauté the minced onion or chives, garlic, celery and green pepper in the remainder of the oil, then add together with the apple, cheese, chopped giblets, herbs, parsley, beaten eggs, salt and sunflower seed meal to the rice, mixing thoroughly. Fill the salted and oiled cavity of the fowl, being careful not to pack too full, since the rice will continue to swell during the roasting period. Wild rice (soaked beforehand according to the directions on the package) makes an even more delicious stuffing. Of course, with the rice stuffing such as this, you'll not serve potatoes or bread, in order to keep the meal predominantly high-protein.

FISH FILETS IN SOUR SAUCE

1 large, or 2 smaller filets per serving (cod, halibut, sole, flounder, whitefish and fresh tuna are some of the types from which to select)
3 tbsp. butter or cooking oil
2¼ cups meat or chicken stock
3 tbsp. millet meal
3 nasturtium seeds, pinch of

1½ tsp. salt
4 tbsp. cooking wine, lemon juice, or wine vinegar
1 small onion, or 2 tbsp. chopped chives or leeks
dill seeds, or chopped sprig of fresh dill
pinch of sweet basil

Remove skin from the filets, rinse well and wipe. Rub salt well into each filet, and allow to stand for about one hour, wiping again. Melt half the fat in a heavy skillet, brown the onion, if used, lightly; but if chives are substituted add them to the sauce a few minutes before removing from the fire. Put the filets in the pan with the hot oil and browned onions. Add half the stock (exact amount will depend upon the quantity of fish prepared) and half the wine or lemon juice. Cover and allow to simmer gently over a low fire for 10 to 15 minutes. Meanwhile, prepare the sauce by heating the balance of the fat in a saucepan, remove from stove, blend in the millet meal to a smooth paste, then gradually stir in the remaining stock. Salt to taste.

Boil for 5 to 8 minutes, stirring until smooth and thickened, then add the remainder of the wine or lemon juice and pour over the filets that have been placed on a hot platter. Sprinkle with paprika and serve with small new potatoes steamed in their jackets, a vegetable salad and a custard pudding.

ITALIAN BAKED FISH WITH STUFFING

1 large baking fish
6 tbsp. cooking oil or melted butter
4 tbsp. chopped chives
1 clove garlic
1 cup whole-grain bread crumbs (or wheat germ or millet meal)
2 tbsp. milk
4 tbsp. grated Romano cheese
4 tbsp. chopped fresh or canned mushrooms
1 tbsp. chopped parsley
1 tbsp. chopped fresh mint, or fresh dill (2 tsp. crushed dill seeds may be used instead)
salt to taste
1 lemon, sliced

Choose any of the following for baked fish: whitefish, large trout, pompano, salmon, red snapper, pickerel, mackerel, halibut, haddock, cod, bluefish, swordfish or shad. Have the fish cleaned, slit down the center, and boned. Rub the inside well with salt and cooking oil. Prepare the stuffing by heating the peeled garlic clove in 3 tablespoons of the oil in a heavy skillet. Remove the garlic if only a mild flavor is desired, otherwise allow to remain in the stuffing. Then sauté the mushrooms and parsley in the garlic-flavored oil for about 15 minutes. Remove from the fire. Using a large mixing bowl, combine the mushrooms with the bread crumbs, milk (stuffing must be slightly moist but not too soft to remain in the fish), herbs, cheese and salt to taste. Stuff the fish, then sew or skewer edges firmly together. Place in an open baking pan in which the remainder of the oil or butter has been melted. Bake in a moderate (350° F.) oven for about 30 to 35 minutes, or until the fish is tender. Remove to a warmed platter, garnish with lemon slices, and serve with a tossed green salad, a cooked green vegetable and a fruit custard.

SAVORY PAN FISH

Allow 2 to 3 pan fish per serving, depending on size
6 tbsp. cooking oil or melted butter
6 to 9 anchovy filets, chopped
1 tsp. fresh mint chopped, or dried mint leaves
1 tsp. chopped parsley
salt to taste
4 tbsp. lemon juice, cooking wine, or wine vinegar

Clean the fish (brook trout, small perch, sunfish, bluegills or other pan fish), and dry well. Then salt to taste. Brown slowly in the fat until almost done, then add the herbs, chopped anchovy filets and cooking wine or lemon juice. Simmer for a few minutes longer until the fish is tender. Serve with baked or steamed-in-the-jacket potatoes, creamed vegetable and a fruit pie.

SHRIMP-IN-A-NEST

3 cups cooked brown rice
4 tbsp. cooking oil or melted butter
1 garlic clove
2 cups cooked fresh shrimp (canned, or boiled frozen shrimp may be used instead)
2 tbsp. chopped green pepper
2 cups cooked peas, or lima beans
2 cups canned tomatoes
½ cup diced celery
1 tsp. sweet basil
salt to taste

Heat the oil with the garlic in a deep saucepan; add the chopped pepper and celery, cooking for 10 to 15 minutes over a low flame. Then stir in the tomatoes, sweet basil and salt. Cook slowly for 20 minutes, stirring occasionally. Add the shrimp, and peas or beans. Cover the saucepan and allow the shrimp to heat through, about 5 minutes. Put a nest of warm cooked brown rice on each plate, then fill the center with the shrimp sauce. This is a dish I discovered in the Bayou country of Louisiana where Cajuns know how to prepare shrimp as no other people can. Like many other recipes I've given you, this is a one-dish meal. Add a fruit salad and a dessert made with milk, and you have a perfectly balanced high-protein meal.

SINGAPORE SHRIMP AND RICE

1½ cups brown rice
3 eggs, well-beaten
1 lb. fresh cooked shrimp, or about 2 cups canned shrimp
2 tbsp. butter
4 tbsp. cooking oil
¼ tsp. curry powder
salt to taste
2 tbsp. chopped parsley
1 tbsp. soy sauce

After washing well, steam the brown rice until each grain stands apart. Drop the shrimp into a skillet with the hot butter, add the soy sauce and curry powder, together with about 2 tablespoons of warm water, blend well and sauté for about 10 minutes. Then make a simple omelet of the beaten eggs, seasoned with salt, and cooked in the oil (allow to cook very slowly on one side before turning, so the omelet comes out in one piece like a large pancake), then cut in narrow strips. Mix the curried shrimp, egg strips and cooked rice together lightly. If the mixture seems a little too dry, blend a little soy sauce through it. Sprinkle with the chopped parsley (or chopped chives). Addition of the eggs makes this an unusually high-protein meatless or Lenten dish.

ARGENTINE TUCO SAUCE

½ lb. chopped beef
4 tbsp. cooking oil
½ small can Italian tomato paste
1 cup cooked sliced mushrooms
1 garlic clove
3 tbsp. grated Italian cheese (Romano or Parmesan)

1 large can plum tomatoes
salt to taste
pinch each of dried sweet marjoram, sweet basil, thyme, powdered cardamon
1 bay leaf
1 whole clove

Sauté the beef in the heated oil in a deep, heavy saucepan, then cover and allow to simmer for about 5 minutes, stirring frequently to prevent sticking. Add the canned plum tomatoes, the herbs, the garlic and the salt, and allow to cook over a very low flame for 45 minutes, stirring occasionally. Then blend in the tomato paste, and continue cooking over the lowest possible fire for about another 30 minutes, stirring frequently to prevent sticking. You'll find that the longer this sauce cooks, the more wonderful its flavor. In fact, if you can prepare it the day before and store in the refrigerator to be reheated immediately before using, so much the better. Immediately before serving stir in the grated cheese. This is the "genuine" Italian spaghetti sauce. Serve it on whole-wheat spaghetti or noodles, or even on corn meal or millet meal polenta (mush flavored with grated cheese). In the Argentine, I ate this "tuco," as it's called in that country, served over *tallarines* (noodles) that were flavored and colored green with finely chopped kale. This made an extremely delicious meal when served with a tossed salad and a bowl of fresh fruits.

MEAT BROTH (BASIC RECIPE)

Never throw away a meat bone, cooked or uncooked, or poultry bones. They're worth real money to you for soups and broths. This holds good also for meat trimmings, or leftover bits of cooked meat. In other words, save all bones, fat and trimmings from meat or poultry. Bring them home with you; don't let the butcher keep what is the foundation of a nourishing broth for your family. Be thrifty! If you're not going to make broth for a day or so, keep the bones and trimmings in the refrigerator, adding to them the cooked bones and unused portions of cooked meats or a chicken carcass. Then when broth day comes, add all your "savings" to about 1 quart of cold water, plus about 1 tablespoon of lemon juice or wine vinegar in order to dissolve the calcium from the bones, as well as to give a piquant flavor to the broth. Bring slowly to a boil, skim off any excess fat, and allow to simmer, covered, for at least an hour, adding ½ teaspoon of salt and whatever herbs are desired for seasoning. A splendid soup seasoning is an herb salt that contains something like 14 different properly blended herbs, plus a good grade of salt. If the meat flavor of the broth is not pronounced enough to suit the taste, add about ¼ to ½ teaspoon of meat extract or a bouillon cube. You can make up this stock and have it in the refrigerator, ready for use at any time, merely by having the forethought to make use of uncooked or leftover bones and meat trimmings as they accumulate. I don't know why it is, but a recipe calling for "stock" usually frightens most cooks away; perhaps because they don't have such an item on hand. But the kitchen-wise cook knows that it's no trick to have stock or broth on hand at all times, for serving plain as a before-meal appetite stimulant, or for incorporating into other delicious soup recipes.

SUNSHINE SOUP (MEATLESS)

4 tbsp. sunflower seed meal
1½ cups consommé
1¼ cups tomato purée
1 cup of shredded carrot
1 clove garlic
4 tbsp. water
2 tbsp. butter

pinch of sweet basil
1 bay leaf
1 cassia bud or 1 small whole clove
pinch of raw or brown sugar
salt to taste

Melt the butter in a deep saucepan, add the carrots and garlic, and sauté lightly for about 2 to 3 minutes. Then add the water, tomato purée, salt, herbs and sugar. Cover the pan, and allow to steam until the carrot is tender. Blend the consommé into the sunflower seed meal, then add to the tomato mixture, allowing to heat for 1 to 2 minutes. Serve, topping each bowl with a heaping tablespoon of yogurt, half moons of avocado, or a sprinkling of chopped green onions. This makes a creamy, highly nutritious protein soup—one that's destined for widespread popularity.

Chapter 24

MEAT SUBSTITUTES THAT ARE PROTEIN

WHENEVER it's necessary for you to seek a substitute dish for meat (which I hope is not too often), for the sake of your long-lasting youth don't turn to the "noodle and spaghetti" section of your cookbook.

As I pointed out to you earlier, *starch can never be a safe substitute for protein.*

Here are some substitute meat dishes which contain high-grade protein, and which can well be adopted into your menu-planning as a means of easing up on your budget. The following recipes, together with the egg and cheese recipes and the seed cereal recipes, are the only *protein* substitutes for meat that you can schedule in a menu with the full assurance that you're not completely shortchanging yourself and your family on *health* for that day.

First we'll take a look at all the delicious ways in which sunflower seeds (a *complete* protein, you'll remember) can be called into service as a pinch hitter for meat.

SUNFLOWER ROAST

1 cup hulled sunflower seeds
1 cup whole-grain bread crumbs (or wheat germ or millet meal)
1 tbsp. sunflower seed meal
1 egg
2 tsp. meat extract paste
5 tbsp. chopped leeks or chives (onion may be used, if tolerated)

3 tsp. chopped parsley
2 tbsp. cooking oil or butter
1 tbsp. lemon juice
pinch each of thyme, sweet marjoram, sweet basil, summer savory, meat or chicken stock, or broth made from soup cubes

Sauté the chopped leeks or chives in the oil or butter. Mix the coarsely ground sunflower seeds with the bread crumbs, herbs and sunflower seed meal. Add the sautéed leeks, well-beaten egg, lemon juice and meat extract which has been melted in enough stock to moisten so the mixture can be molded into a firm loaf. Place in a greased loaf pan, dot with pieces of butter or sprinkle with grated cheese. Bake in a moderate oven (350° F.) 40 to 50 minutes, or until the center of the roast is done. Serve with a tomato or brown sauce. This meat substitute saw hundreds of Britons through their "austerity days" of little or no meat. It makes a tasty, nutlike loaf that is equally good hot or cold. Try serving it with a tossed green salad and a fruit dessert.

SUNSHINE BURGER

1 cup of sunflower seed meal
3 finely grated carrots
½ cup chopped celery
2 tbsp. finely chopped onion or leeks (optional)
1 tsp. chopped parsley
1 tbsp. cooking oil or melted butter
salt to taste
¼ cup milk (garlic-flavored)
pinch of sweet basil

Combine all the ingredients with enough of the milk so they may be molded into patties about ½-inch thick. Place in a shallow oiled baking pan, and bake until brown on both sides. These patties are good either hot or cold, and make a good protein food for a lunch box. While hot they may be served with a butter sauce. For variety add 2 tablespoons chopped ripe or stuffed olives, and 1 tablespoon grated Italian cheese.

SUNFLOWER PEPPERS

4 large green peppers for stuffing (tomatoes, sweet onions, or fresh red pimentoes may also be used)
⅓ cup whole-grain bread crumbs (or wheat germ or millet meal)
½ cup coarsely chopped sunflower seed kernels
⅓ cup grated cheese, Italian or American
1 tbsp. cooking oil or melted butter
⅓ cup tomato juice
2 tsp. chopped parsley
2 tsp. finely chopped onions, leeks, or chives
salt to taste
pinch of sweet basil
¾ cup meatless stock made from Vegex or bouillon cubes (beef extract may also be used)

Prepare the peppers for stuffing by cutting off stem end and removing seeds and pulp. Mix together the bread crumbs, chopped sunflower seed kernels, 4 tablespoons of the grated cheese, oil, parsley, onion and seasonings, adding a little of the stock, if needed, to make a firm mixture. Fill the peppers with the mixture, allowing it to pile up on top. Place in a greased casserole. Mix the remaining stock and the tomato juice, and pour around the peppers. Cover and bake in a moderate oven (350° F.) for about 40 to 50 minutes, or until the peppers are tender. Baste them occasionally with the liquid. Remove the cover during the last 10 minutes and sprinkle the top of each pepper with the remaining cheese. Allow the cheese to melt. Serve with the liquid, plain or slightly thickened, as a sauce. The peppers for this oven dish may be stuffed the night before, or early in the morning, and placed in the refrigerator until time to add the liquid and bake. This makes an easily prepared, nourishing entrée for a busy day.

CONGEE

Anyone who has traveled in the Far East will recognize this as the "hash" of the Oriental kitchen. When prepared with millet meal it yields a dish of high-protein value, exclusive of the meat or fowl it contains. Instead of leftover meats, bits of cooked fish or anchovy filets may be substituted, together with sliced hardcooked eggs. In fact, congee is a delicious, economical, highly nourishing dish.

Prepare millet meal porridge. After the millet has come to a first boil, add the leftover meat, fowl, or cooked fish, and about 1 scant teaspoon of Vegex or beef extract. Allow to cook in a double boiler over boiling water for about 30 minutes longer. Congee may be served immediately, or allowed to remain in the refrigerator for several days and then reheated. In fact, the flavor is more pronounced the second day. In order to warm it over, it may be necessary to thin with a little broth or stock. After removing from the fire, add a little chopped parsley and a few drops of lemon juice. Serve with chopped green onions, chopped chives or sprinkled with chopped fresh dill. Any chopped cooked vegetable may be added.

If you are a vegetarian, prepare your congee by stirring in ½ cup grated American cheese while the millet porridge is still hot, instead of the meat or fowl, and serve as described. Avoid overheating the cheese, otherwise it will become stringy. Congee may also be cooked with onion and served with cooked fish, anchovy filets or scrambled eggs.

MILLET LOAF

4 heaping tbsp. *hulled* millet seed

1 tbsp. chopped onion, leeks or chives

1 cup water
1 small can peas
1 tsp. Vegex or beef extract
2 tbsp. cooking oil or butter
2 cups shredded carrots
2 eggs, beaten
1 tbsp. raw sugar or honey

pinch of sweet basil and thyme
sprig of fresh dill chopped, or ⅛ tsp. crushed dill seeds
salt to taste
2 tbsp. grated cheese
1 tbsp. tomato paste

Soak the millet seed in 1 cup of cold water for several hours, drain, and steam with the juice from the peas and the Vegex or beef extract until the seeds are done. Add the mashed peas, carrots, beaten egg, tomato paste, onion, fat and seasonings. Blend well, form into a loaf, place in a greased loaf pan, and allow to bake in a slow oven (300° to 325° F.) for 45 to 60 minutes. About 10 minutes before removing from the oven, sprinkle the top of the loaf with the grated cheese and allow to melt. Serve with a green salad bowl and a fruit dessert.

ALMOND-MILLET LOAF

½ cup cold, thickened millet porridge
½ cup almonds, finely ground
½ cup grated coconut

2 tbsp. wheat germ
1 tsp. herb flavored salt
1 cup canned tomatoes

Blend into a smooth mixture, shape into a loaf and place in a greased pan. Bake in a slow oven (300° to 325° F.) until nicely browned. This is something different in the way of a meatless loaf; it can be used to add taste variety to meatless menus. If desired, chopped olives, raisins or red pimentos may also be added. Serve with a cooked green vegetable, a tossed or finger salad, and a dessert containing eggs and milk.

SEED NUT LOAF

⅓ cup hulled sunflower seeds, finely chopped
⅓ cup sesame seed meal
⅓ cup walnuts or almonds, finely chopped
1½ cups cooked lima beans, mashed
1½ cups cooked carrots, chopped
2 tbsp. minced onion or chives

3 eggs, lightly beaten
1½ tbsp. cooking oil or melted butter
1½ cups non-fat milk
1½ cups soft whole-grain bread crumbs (or wheat germ or millet meal)
salt to taste
dash of paprika
2 tsp. lemon juice

Add the milk and lightly beaten eggs to the crumbs and combine all ingredients. Pack into a well-greased loaf pan. Bake in a moderate oven (350° F.) for 45 minutes, or until firm. Serve with tomato, cream or mushroom sauce. This is a valuable high-protein loaf that can safely take the place of meat or fowl in a meal. Serve with a tossed green salad, a cube of cheese and a fruit cup.

TAMALE LOAF

1 cup millet meal, or yellow unbolted cornmeal	4 tbsp. grated Italian cheese (Parmesan or Romano)
1 small can mushrooms, or 1 pint fresh mushrooms	¾ cup grated Cheddar cheese
4 tbsp. cooking oil	2⅓ cups canned tomatoes
1 tbsp. minced onion (optional)	3 cups hot water
1 clove garlic	½ cup cold water
	1 tsp. salt
	pinch of sweet basil and sweet marjoram

Sauté the onions (if used) in the heated oil, add the mushrooms and sauté lightly, then stir in the tomatoes, half of the salt and the garlic. Allow to simmer very slowly for about 1½ hours, stirring frequently to prevent sticking. (The garlic clove may be removed after the first 30 minutes, if only a mild flavor is desired.) Then prepare the mush by mixing the meal with the cold water, and adding gradually to the salted boiling water, stirring until the mush thickens and bubbles to a boil. Lower the flame and cook over a slow fire for about 12 minutes longer. Place a layer of the mush in the bottom of a greased shallow casserole or baking dish, cover with a layer of the tomato-mushroom sauce, add a third layer of the grated Cheddar cheese, and repeat, ending up with a topping of the mush sprinkled with the grated Italian cheese, making sure to save some of the sauce to serve over the tamale loaf. Bake uncovered in a slow oven (300° to 325° F.) for about 30 minutes. Serve with a tossed green salad, and for dessert add an orange custard.

EGGPLANT STEAKS

1 large eggplant (firm, glossy and dark purple)	pinch of salt
	cooking oil or melted butter
4 eggs, well-beaten	
¼ cup grated Romano cheese	1 garlic clove

Peel the eggplant, slice into ¼ inch "steaks" and sprinkle *very lightly* with salt. Pile one slice on top of the other, cover with a heavy plate and allow to stand for 1 hour in order to extract the acrid juices which cause some persons to dislike this valuable member of the vegetable kingdom. Rinse thoroughly with clean water, then dry each slice thoroughly. Make a batter of the eggs, cheese and salt. Dip the eggplant steaks into this batter and drop into a heavy skillet containing the heated shortening in which the clove of garlic has been lightly browned. (If you keep a jar of garlic oil on hand, this will not be necessary.) Allow each side of the steaks to cook over a medium flame for about 5 minutes, or until golden brown. Serve hot with a green salad bowl, a portion of cottage cheese and a fruit pudding or sherbet.

CHEESE NUT LOAF

1 cup chopped walnuts

4 tbsp. sunflower seed meal, sesame seed meal or a mixture of both

1½ cups grated American cheese

1 cup dry whole-wheat bread crumbs (or wheat germ or millet meal)

2 eggs, well-beaten

2 tbsp. chopped chives, or 1 tsp. minced onion

⅓ cup milk

4 tsp. cooking oil or melted butter

2 tbsp. lemon juice
dash of mace or nutmeg
salt to taste

If onions are used, brown lightly in the fat, add the milk, then blend into the bread crumbs. Stir in the well-beaten eggs, add the grated cheese, nuts, seed meal, lemon juice, chives and seasonings. Mix well. If too stiff add enough more milk to form a molded loaf. Pack into a greased loaf pan, top with a few of the bread crumbs held in reserve, dot with butter and bake in a slow oven (300° to 325° F.) for 30 to 40 minutes. This makes a nutritious, satisfying entrée, and should be served with a cooked green vegetable, a green salad and a fruit dessert.

Now, after reading through this far-from-complete listing of "meat substitutes that are protein," don't you agree that it's purely lack of imagination, at the best, which causes a housewife or a home economist to turn to the high-starch, low-nutrition macaroni and rice dishes for meatless menus? With a little ingenuity and experimentation, you can concoct other delicious high-protein meat substitutes from adaptations of those I have given you as a starter.

Chapter 25

EGG AND CHEESE DISHES FOR EVERY MEAL

TOGETHER with the meatless dishes listed above, these egg and cheese dishes are splendid menu-extenders and budget-easers. In addition, they are high protein, tasty and offer variety to the menu. Especially will you find many new and different ideas for high-protein breakfast main dishes among them.

These egg and cheese dishes may be served also at luncheon or dinner. In fact, if the midday meal is a substantial meat one, then I recommend that a light egg or cheese entrée be served for supper in the case of persons whose physical activities are no longer strenuous enough to demand a heartier evening meal. Moreover, these egg and cheese dishes provide excellent entrées for the invalid's tray, or for the meals planned for elderly persons.

COTTAGE CHEESE OMELET

4 eggs, well-beaten	1 tbsp. skim milk powder
4 heaping tbsp. cottage cheese	dash of salt
	sprinkle of paprika
	pinch of sweet basil

Beat the cottage cheese until creamy, stir in the milk powder, blending until perfectly smooth. Season and add the very well-beaten eggs. (For a fluffier omelet, beat egg yolks and white separately, folding in the stiffly beaten whites at the very last.) Pour into a buttered omelet pan or heavy skillet and cook over very low heat until lightly browned. If an omelet pan is not used, the omelet must either be turned like a pancake, or allowed to finish cooking in a moderate oven (350° F.) after the bottom is lightly browned.

EGGS HAWAIIAN

1 egg per person	1 tsp. grated fresh or un-sweetened coconut per egg
1 tsp. yogurt per egg	salt to taste
1 tsp. powdered skim milk per egg	

I'm about to let you in one the taste secret that makes scrambled eggs at the Royal Hawaiian Hotel in Honolulu an experience not to be forgotten. Like everything else superb in the culinary world, the secret lies in a simple little taste trick —coconut! Scramble the eggs in the usual way by beating well, then blending in the cream, milk powder and salt. Add the coconut, and turn into a well-buttered skillet over a very low flame, allowing the under layer to set well before lifting the edges so the uncooked top portion may run down. Watch closely to avoid overcooking. If preferred, the eggs may be scrambled in a double boiler, a method which requires no butter and is an excellent way to prepare scrambled eggs for a reducing diet.

EGGS A LA SICILIANA

4 eggs (1 per person)
4 chicken livers
1 tbsp. tomato paste
1 tbsp. chopped onion, leeks or chives

3 tbsp. cooking oil
4 tbsp. warm water
4 tbsp. cooking wine
salt to taste

Sauté the halved chicken livers and the onions in the heated oil for about 5 minutes over a slow fire. Add the tomato paste which has been diluted by the warm water. Salt to taste, and allow to simmer slowly for 5 minutes. Add the wine and continue cooking for 3 minutes. Then, one at a time in order not to break the yolks, slip in the eggs. Cover the pan and allow the eggs to poach for 3 minutes, or until the whites are firm. Serve at once. This is my favorite version of poached eggs.

"101 WAYS" TO SCRAMBLE EGGS

Allowing 1 to 2 eggs per person, add 1 tablespoon of top milk, cream or sour cream to each egg, plus 2 teaspoons of powdered milk, and prepare the basic scrambled eggs by beating the other ingredients into the eggs until smoothly blended. From there, go on with any of these tasty variations:

2 teaspoons of grated Italian or American cheese per egg
1 teaspoon chopped chives, leeks, fresh dill, diced pimento or minced parsley per egg
1 teaspoon sesame seeds or sunflower seeds per egg
Leftover meat, fish or poultry finely chopped
Flaked smoked fish such as kippers or chubs
Fresh or canned mushrooms

Chopped cooked green vegetables such as broccoli, kale or asparagus

1 teaspoon shredded pineapple (if canned, drain well) per egg

½ teaspoon tomato paste per egg, plus grated Italian or American cheese

Chopped green or ripe olives

Diced avocado added to the pan just before the eggs set well

1 teaspoon of capers per egg

Fresh or cooked fruit (well-drained) such as berries, cooked apple slices, cooked apricots, peaches, prunes or figs

For herb seasonings, try singly, or blended, a pinch of sweet basil, thyme, sweet marjoram, celery seed, rosemary, summer savory or tarragon. An herb salt containing a blend of most of these herbs, plus several others, is sold in most health food stores.

HUNGARIAN EGGS

5 hard-cooked eggs
4 tbsp. grated cheese
1 cup yogurt

1 tbsp. minced parsley
dash of paprika
pinch of sweet basil
salt to taste
2 tsp. chopped chives (optional)

Cut the hard-cooked eggs in half lengthwise. Remove the yolks carefully in order not to tear the white. Using a fork, cream the yolks until smooth, then mix in 3 tablespoons of the yogurt, half the grated cheese and the seasonings. Refill the center of each egg as for deviled eggs, rejoin the halves firmly. Place in a shallow greased dish. Pour the remainder of the sour cream over them, sprinkle with the grated cheese and color with paprika. Allow to brown in the broiler under a very low flame. This savory egg dish is really very simple to prepare since the eggs may be boiled the night before, and they will brown in the broiler while the coffee is perking. This is also a nourishing high-protein dish to pack in a waxed container (a cottage cheese carton, for instance) for the lunch box or picnic basket.

CAMP-STYLE EGGS

6 well-beaten eggs

3 tbsp. chopped chives

½ cup cottage cheese

4 oz. dried beef (approximately 1 cup of dried beef pulled into pieces)

2 tbsp. cooking oil or butter

(onion may be used instead)

(go easy on the salt, remember the dried beef is already salty!)

Sauté the dried beef in the fat over a low flame with the chives or onions. Beat the eggs as for an omelet, then add the cottage cheese and continue beating until well blended and smooth. Pour this mixture over the sautéed beef and allow to cook over a very low fire until thick and soft, stirring frequently. Garnish with chopped parsley or sprigs of fresh dill. For high-protein content, this dish can't be beat. It contains three high-protein items—eggs, cottage cheese and meat. And, besides, it's so darned good! This is one version of scrambled eggs that will make a big hit with the men of the family.

EGGS FOO YUNG

4 eggs

1 No. 2 can bean sprouts (1 lb. of fresh sprouts)

2 green peppers

1 small onion

½ cup cooked beef, lamb, chicken, shrimp or flaked fish

½ tsp. salt

1 tbsp. powdered skim milk

The meat, peppers and onion must either be finely chopped or put through the food grinder. Add the bean sprouts. In a separate bowl beat the eggs as for an omelet or scrambled eggs. Blend in the meat and vegetables, and salt. Drop from a tablespoon onto a hot oiled griddle as for pancakes, and allow to brown lightly on both sides. Serve with soy sauce and brown rice. Chopped celery may be used instead of bean sprouts. Mushrooms and sliced water chestnuts also make tasty additions to this typically Chinese dish. Eggs Foo Yung may be served at any meal for a nourishing entrée that does not leave you with a stuffed feeling. Try it for Sunday morning breakfast instead of the proverbial "waffles and sausage."

SERBIAN CHEESE

2 cups cottage cheese

2 tbsp. minced green pepper

2 tbsp. minced chives

2 tsp. celery seed

1 tsp. celery salt

1 tbsp. finely chopped sweet pickles

2 tbsp. chopped pimentos

Cream the cheese until smooth, adding a little sweet or sour cream if necessary. Add the other ingredients and blend well. Chill for several hours, then serve either as a salad, a sandwich spread or the entrée for a warm weather luncheon or light supper.

COTTAGE CHEESE VARIATIONS

Cottage cheese, that wonderful high-protein food which is so kind to your budget (and to your figure), may be seasoned in a number of appetizing ways. Here are only a few of the possible variations. You'll enjoy experimenting to find others that please your household!

Into each cup of cottage cheese blend 2 tablespoons of crushed caraway seeds, and season with salt.

Chopped chives, leeks, onions or a bit of garlic flavoring give the bland cheese that savory taste which assures a successful salad or sandwich filling.

Chopped fresh dill or crushed dill seeds added to the cottage cheese make a flavorful salad to be served with fish dishes.

Chopped cooked chicken, or other fowl, plus ½ teaspoon of lemon juice to 1 cup of cottage cheese makes a delicious salad or entrée for luncheon, a light supper, or even for a different breakfast dish.

A little honey blended into cottage cheese, together with peanut butter, sesame seed butter, or sunflower seed meal makes a sandwich filling far superior to the unimaginative all-sweet jelly filling which finds its way all too frequently into the lunch box of school children or working persons.

Use whipped cottage cheese as a dressing for a green salad containing tomatoes, in place of high-calorie oil dressings.

For a breakfast dish that is light and tasty, serve whipped cottage cheese over fresh or cooked fruits, or berries.

Mix 1 tablespoon of yogurt into each cup of cottage cheese. Add about ⅛ teaspoon of honey and a dash of cinnamon. This is a favorite dessert in Middle European countries.

PORTUGUESE CHEESE

2 cups cottage cheese, whipped

6 anchovy filets chopped very fine, or 1 tbsp. anchovy paste

1 tbsp. crushed caraway seeds

1 tbsp. minced capers

1 tbsp. minced chives

⅛ tsp. dry mustard (optional)

2 tsp. paprika

Whip the cottage cheese until smooth, adding a little sweet or sour cream if necessary. Blend in the chopped anchovy filets or the paste, then add the other ingredients, reserving the paprika to be sprinkled over the molded mound of cheese. Set in the refrigerator to chill for an hour or so, and serve on a bed of salad greens with garnishes of lemon slices. I first tasted this wonderful cheese in Rio de Janerio where it was served to me in the home of an aristocratic old Portuguese family. The recipe had been brought to Brazil from Portugal in the early nineteenth century when the Brazilian dynasty was founded.

COTTAGE CHEESE PANCAKES

1 cup moist cottage cheese (if dry, add a little milk or yogurt to moisten)
2 eggs well-beaten
1½ tsp. honey, raw sugar

½ cup whole-wheat flour
½ tsp. baking powder
½ tsp. salt
1 tsp. grated lemon rind
dash of nutmeg

Sift together the dry ingredients. Add the well-beaten eggs to which have been added the cheese, lemon rind, nutmeg and honey or sugar. Bake on a hot greased griddle, and serve with a teaspoon of yogurt or a little honey or syrup on each pancake. This is truly a high-protein pancake. You'll like these for either breakfast or a light supper.

UKRAINIAN CHEESE CAKES

2 cups dry cottage cheese
2 tbsp. yogurt
2 eggs, well-beaten
1 tbsp. honey

½ tsp. salt
2 tbsp. whole-wheat flour
2 tbsp. butter
6 tbsp. finely ground hazelnuts

Rub the dry cottage cheese through a sieve, or force through a potato ricer. Blend into it the other ingredients, mixing well. Form into flat cakes about 2 inches wide, and sauté in melted butter until golden brown on both sides. Serve with cold sour cream, or top with raw sugar and a dash of cinnamon and a little grated lemon peel. These wonderful cheese cakes provide a novel breakfast dish to replace the old soggy white-flour pancake or waffle. Ground almonds, sunflower seed kernels or sunflower seed meal may be substituted for the hazelnuts with equally delicious results.

MANCHURIAN MILLET SOUFFLÉ

1½ cups cooked hulled millet seed, or millet meal mush
¾ cup grated Cheddar cheese

⅔ cup non-fat milk
3 eggs
grated rind of half a lemon
salt to taste

Separate the eggs, and beat the yolks until thick and lemon-colored, and the whites until stiff enough to stand in little peaks, but not too dry. Add the millet, milk and seasonings to the egg yolks; then the cheese, reserving about ¼ cup as a topping. Fold in last the stiffly beaten whites and pour at once into a greased casserole that will fit into a larger pan of hot water. Sprinkle the remainder of the cheese across the top and set the pan of hot water containing the casserole in a moderate oven (350° F.) until the soufflé sets. This should take from 20 to 25 minutes. Serve at once, adding a tomato salad, a cooked green vegetable and a fruit dessert.

POLISH SOUFFLE

Prepare a thick hot millet mush by moistening 1 cup of millet meal with ¼ cup of cold water, then stirring slowly into a scant 3 cups of boiling salted water. Allow to cook in the top of a double boiler for 20 to 30 minutes, or until thick. Stir frequently. When done, cover the bottom of a shallow greased baking dish with half the hot mush. Spread with 1¼ cups of shredded snappy cheese, and cover with the remaining mush. Pour 1¼ cups of yogurt or whipped cottage cheese over the top and bake in a 375° to 400° F. oven for 10 to 15 minutes. Serve hot with a cooked green vegetable, a tossed salad, and a fruit cup.

By no means do the recipes above comprise all the nourishing, appetizing and "different" ways of serving eggs and cheese. But with these few recipes as a guide, I'm hoping you'll no longer fall into the rut of serving all eggs either fried or boiled, and all cheese in a sandwich! Eggs and cheese are two of your most valuable high-protein foods. Use them often—and use your imagination to keep them from showing up on the table in the same old monotonous ways.

Chapter 26

EAT PLENTY OF SEED CEREALS

SEED and whole-grain cereals, and the porridges and various tasty dishes that may be made with them, have a definite place in everyone's diet regardless of age, but especially in the diets of those past forty, since the B-vitamins and high-grade proteins supplied by these seed and whole-grain cereals are needed more and more as the years slip by. Throw out any dry or devitalized cereal on your pantry shelf, and convert at once to seed or whole-grain cereals. All those artificial, patented cereals are nothing more nor less than 100 per cent starch.

When you prepare the mush or porridges shown below, allow for some to be left over, since it may be served in a number of delicious, nourishing ways, either for breakfast, lunch or a light supper.

MILLET MEAL PORRIDGE

1 cup millet meal or *hulled* millet seed

3½ to 4 cups of water (or half milk and half water)

¼ tsp. honey or raw sugar salt to taste

Use less water for a thick mush, and more for porridge. Mix the millet meal and salt with 1 cup of the cold liquid in the top of a double boiler until the meal is smoothly blended into a paste, then add the remainder of the liquid (boiling if water is used, or scalded if milk). Place over boiling water, cover and allow to cook slowly for 20 to 30 minutes, stirring frequently to prevent lumping or sticking. A few minutes before taking from the fire, stir in ¼ teaspoon of honey, or raw sugar. This will not sweeten enough to suit some palates, but it does bring out the flavor of the meal, and I find it makes a more tasty cooked cereal to add this small amount of sweetening at this particular time in the cooking. Serve with warmed milk or douse with a mixture of honey and melted butter heated together as for pancakes or waffles. It's entirely out of balance to serve toast with any breakfast that includes a seed cereal either prepared as a porridge or mush.

For variety when the meal is cooked to a thin porridge, stir in dried fruits such as sliced dates, figs, apricots, prunes or raisins when it is about half-cooked. Or each serving may be topped with fresh or cooked peaches, pineapple, berries or other fruits. Serve with fresh fruits such as bananas, peaches or berries by placing the fruits in the bottom of the cereal bowl, and in alternate layers with the cereal, sprinkling raw sugar or honey over each layer of the fruit, and covering with milk if desired.

For a full-bodied mush, omit the honey or raw sugar and stir in about ⅓ cup of grated American, Cheddar or Italian cheese such as Romano or Parmesan after removing the cereal from the fire. When this mixture hardens it may be sliced and sautéed to make a delicious cheese mush.

Stir in one heaping tablespoon of sunflower seed or sesame seed meal as the mush or porridge is taken from the fire. This gives added flavor and extra protein to your breakfast cereal.

MILLET MUSH PATTIES

Pack leftover or specially prepared millet meal mush into a square or rectangular mold (a loaf pan) rinsed with cold water. Chill until firm. Remove from the mold in a solid cake, and slice about ¼ to ½ inch thick. Dip each slice in an egg batter and drop into a heavy skillet containing hot butter, margarine or cooking oil. Allow each side to brown to a delicious golden shade. Serve piping hot with butter and honey. This is especially fine for Sunday morning breakfast.

MILLET SCRAPPLE

When the millet mush is about half-cooked, add small pieces of cooked meat, fowl or fish. Season with a pinch of thyme, sweet marjoram and sweet basil; or use an herb salt containing these and other properly blended herbs. Press down into a loaf pan rinsed in cold water, and cover to prevent a crust from forming. Chill overnight. When ready to use, cut in ¼ to ½ inch slices and sauté in melted butter or garlic oil until crisp and nicely browned on both sides. The slices may be dipped in millet or fine whole-grain bread crumbs, then in a slightly beaten egg, and back into the millet meal or crumbs again before sautéeing. This gives the scrapple a deliciously brown crust. I know of no heartier high-protein main breakfast dish on a cold morning than this millet scrapple.

For variety, add finely chopped sunflower seed kernels, browned sesame seeds, or chopped blanched almonds to the mush instead of meat, and season with 1 teaspoon of raw sugar or honey, and several drops of lemon juice.

DOUBLE-BOILER MILLET BREAD

1 cup whole-grain flour
¾ cup millet meal
¼ cup unbolted yellow corn-meal
2½ tsp. baking powder
1 tsp. salt

2 tbsp. honey, raw or brown sugar
½ lb. pitted dates, chopped; or ¾ cup seedless raisins
1½ cups fortified non-fat milk
2 tbsp. melted butter or cooking oil

Mix and sift the dry ingredients. Stir in the dates or raisins. Add the milk, then the melted shortening, stirring only enough to mix well. Turn into the top of a well-greased double boiler, cover and cook over boiling water for approximately 2 hours. Slice and serve hot with butter, cream cheese or yogurt thickened with a little honey. This makes about 8 large slices. It is an economical, easy-to-make high-protein bread.

CALIFORNIA SPOON BREAD

1 cup unbolted yellow corn-meal
½ cup millet meal, sunflower seed meal, or mixed
1 tsp. salt
2¼ tsp. baking powder

1 cup fortified milk
1 cup buttermilk, yogurt or sour milk
3 eggs, separated
1 tbsp. honey, or raw sugar

Sift the meals and salt together and scald with just enough boiling water to wet thoroughly without making it soft and mushy. Allow to cool. Then add the two combined milks a little at a time. Beat in the already well-beaten yolks and the sugar or honey, and baking powder. Blend well into the batter. Fold in last the stiffly beaten whites. Pour into a greased casserole or deep baking dish. Bake in a moderately hot oven (350° to 375° F.) for about 40 to 45 minutes, or until the custard is set and a nicely browned crust is formed. Serve at once from the baking dish, spooning out the portions, to be doused with plain butter, or butter and honey (maple syrup is good, too). Because this is a "spoon bread," the texture will resemble that of a thick custard, for that is exactly what it is, a meal custard—and a most delicious one, I might add. Serve it for Sunday breakfast, for lunch, or for light suppers. It's a protein meal in itself.

Chapter 27

SALADS ARE IMPORTANT IN YOUR MENUS

WHY salads on American tables and in American restaurants should have degenerated, for the most part, into a dispirited leaf of lettuce underlying a slice or two of anemic tomato and topped by a splash of unappetizing-looking dressing I cannot say, unless it be owing to the inertia and "don't-care" of our cooks.

Salads should be the acme of taste thrills in a meal.

The success of your salad lies in two things: (1) the freshness and crispness of the greens, and (2) the kind of dressing you select. Try improving the salads you serve, not only for the sake of better meals, but for the sake of your efforts to build the kind of health that will carry your body youthfully toward a long and active life. When you reach the point in your mealtime planning where, to sit down at lunch or dinner without a nourishing salad, would be like trying to eat a meal without food on your plate, then you will have attained a high degree of nutritional wisdom!

GREEN SALAD BOWL

Lettuce, escarole, chicory, romaine, Chinese cabbage, endive, watercress and dandelion greens are some of the more commonly used salad greens. Wash them thoroughly and allow to drain. Then tear into bite-size pieces with the fingers (never bruise your salad greens by cutting them with a knife), cover and place in the refrigerator until time to serve. The first secret of a tasty green salad is to have all ingredients crisp and chilled, adding the dressing at the last minute. Otherwise the greens are limp and oil-soaked by the time they reach the table. Another taste trick in successful salad preparation is to salt your greens and add the lemon juice or wine vinegar *before* the oil, then toss vigorously. A few suggested green salad combinations are:

Lettuce and watercress
Escarole, tomato quarters, or strips of canned red pimentos and anchovy filets
Lettuce, watercress, romaine, sliced green peppers and tomatoes

198

Lettuce, sliced cucumbers, radishes, chopped chives, green pepper rings

Curly endive, chopped pimento, chopped ripe olives

Escarole, chopped fresh dill, and sliced hard-cooked eggs

Romaine, watercress, and avocado

Mustard greens, watercress, and lettuce, with leaves of fresh summer savory, sweet basil, marjoram and rosemary.

Garlic is the Taste King of a green salad. But so few persons understand the secret of delicacy in the use of garlic seasoning. If you like your salads strongly flavored with garlic, then mince a clove of garlic into the greens. But if you wish to avoid the "social consequences" of a garlic breath, you'll welcome the news that the smell of garlic does not cling to the breath unless the garlic clove is actually swallowed. Therefore, by dropping a peeled clove of garlic into a jar containing about 1½ cups of salad oil and allowing it to "steep" for several hours, even overnight, you may have your garlic-flavored salads and a sweet breath, too.

Keep a jar of this garlic-oil always on hand in the kitchen. Use it for your salads, for sautéeing meats, making stews and flavoring roasts and steaks. If onions do not agree with you, and you still like a pronounced flavor to your salads, soups, meats, gravies and sauces, learn to use garlic without actually eating it, thereby removing the only objection to this splendid cooking herb—its after-effect on the breath. Just remember not to eat the clove itself, and you'll be safe from that unpleasant lingering odor.

FRUIT SALADS

Fresh or canned fruits, berries and melons may be used in numerous combinations to make delicious salads. By omitting the dressing and serving as a dessert instead of on greens, the same combinations make a fruit cup.) Keep an assortment of canned and dried fruits in your cupboard at all times so that you may always have the makings of a fruit salad or fruit cup, even when the supply of fresh fruits in the market is limited, or too costly.

Also keep on hand for salads a good quality of dried apricots, figs, apple rings, pears, peaches and prunes. (Also a few of each of these dried fruits cooked together with a couple of tablespoons of honey and several lemon slices make a delicious breakfast compote.) Honeyed dates (not the pitted, imported variety) blend nicely with most fruit salads, as do nuts, sunflower seed kernels and sesame seed meal.

Recommended fresh fruits for salads are cantaloupe or watermelon balls, berries of all kinds, oranges, tangerine and grapefruit segments, ripe banana slices, apples, pears, peaches, plums, cranberries, nectarines, avocado, grapes and persimmons. Blend any two or more of these canned, fresh or cooked dried fruits as your fancy suggests. Squeeze a few drops of lemon or lime juice over the fruits as soon as blended. Cover and place in the refrigerator until time to serve in order to prevent undue loss of vitamin C through exposure to light and air.

VEGETABLE SALAD

This type of salad is usually a combination of fresh cooked vegetables served on a bed of greens. Again the possibilities for variety are unlimited. Moreover, by combining several vegetables in a salad, you eliminate the need for separate servings of vegetables at a meal. The busy housewife welcomes the two-or-three-dish meal. What's more, she welcomes an opportunity to use up that spoonful or two of this and that vegetable left over from a previous meal. A good combination vegetable salad is the answer, dressed up with one or two fresh vegetables or hard-cooked egg slices.

GOURMET'S SALAD (Serves 6 to 8)

½ head escarole	¼ cup chopped chives
½ head lettuce	1 small cucumber
¼ head endive	Roquefort cheese dressing

Combine the greens, chives and thinly sliced cucumber (do not peel) in a large salad bowl. Immediately before serving toss with Roquefort cheese dressing. Add a slice of cold roast beef, lamb or fowl, and a fruit pudding to this salad, and you have a high-protein meal fit for a king!

SUNFLOWER SALAD

Allow 1 tablespoon of sunflower seed meal for each portion. Prepare a Russian salad by combining diced celery, cooked peas, finely shredded salad greens, quartered ripe tomatoes, cooked and well-drained beets cut in cubes, and finely chopped sweet onion or chopped chives. Blend the vegetables with ½ teaspoon of herb salt and the sunflower seed meal. Add enough Yogurt Dressing to coat the vegetables well when lightly tossed. Arrange a mound of the salad on a salad plate, place strips of raw carrots around it to resemble sunflower petals, garnish the center of the mound with several sunflower seed kernels and crisp green lettuce leaves placed to resemble sunflower leaves. This makes a highly nutritious protein salad that can be made as attractive to the eye as to the taste buds. Serve with a meat soup, a portion of plain cottage cheese and fruit custard for a complete meal.

ALL-IN-ONE PROTEIN SALAD

1 head bibb lettuce, or romaine
2 ripe tomatoes, quartered
1 stalk of green celery, thinly sliced
1 ripe avocado, cut in crescents
2 tbsp. chopped sweet or green onion, or chives
½ cup shredded cold meat, or fowl, or flaked cooked fish

¼ cup crumbled cheese (Roquefort, Gorgonzola, sharp Cheddar are the best, but dry cottage cheese may also be used)
1 sliced hard-cooked egg salt to taste
Sweet Basil Dressing (see recipe)

Wash the greens, drain well, tear into bite-size pieces, cover and place in the refrigerator until time to serve. Combine the meat and vegetables, and toss well with the Sweet Basil Dressing. Chill. When ready to serve, toss this combination, plus the crumbled cheese, lightly with the greens. This salad is an unusually delicious high-energy protein entrée in itself, and is especially recommended for luncheon. During warm weather, serve it with a jellied consommé and a fruit milk sherbet; in cooler weather add a hot broth and a fruit pudding.

SALAD DRESSINGS

With a wide variety of salad dressings, the same tossed salad ingredients can take on new flavor thrills at each serving. Even plain lettuce, often the only salad green available in some communities, may be made into a number of different delicious salads merely by varying the dressing used. Each of the following salad dressing recipes is easy to make, and contains health-building ingredients.

YOGURT DRESSING

1 cup yogurt
1 tsp. lemon juice
¼ tsp. honey

½ tsp. salt
1 tsp. minced chives
⅛ tsp. paprika

Chill yogurt thoroughly. Whip in the honey, salt and chives, adding the lemon juice and paprika last. This makes a little over 1 cup of a nutritious salad dressing. For variety, the finely chopped or sieved yolks of 2 hard-cooked eggs may be added to this yogurt dressing. Keep in the refrigerator. To prepare Garlic Dressing for cooked vegetable salads, omit the honey and allow a split clove of garlic to lie in the yogurt for about 1 hour before preparing the dressing.

FRENCH CREAM DRESSING

½ cup yogurt
¼ cup tomato ketchup
4 tbsp. lemon juice, or 2 tbsp. wine vinegar
½ cup salad oil

½ tsp. salt
2 tsp. honey
¼ tsp. paprika
⅛ tsp. dry mustard (optional)
1 clove garlic

Peel and halve the garlic, allowing it to stand in either the oil or the yogurt for at least 1 to 2 hours before preparing the dressing. Whip the chilled cream, continuing to blend in all the ingredients until thoroughly mixed, starting with the oil, next the tomato ketchup, then the seasonings. Chill before using. Keep in the bottom of the refrigerator as far from the freezing unit as possible otherwise the oil may solidify.

HONEY DRESSING

A delicious dressing for fruit salads is made by using equal parts of olive oil and honey, seasoned with lemon, lime or grapefruit juice to taste, plus a dash of salt. Mix the oil, salt and citrus juice, then slowly beat in the honey, blending well.

FRUIT SALAD DRESSING

1 avocado
¼ cup cream
1 cup orange juice

1 tsp. honey
herb salt to taste

Blend the crushed avocado pulp with the cream. Add the

orange juice and whip with a rotary egg beater until very smooth. Add the honey and salt, and continue beating until slightly thickened. Chill before using. This makes an extremely delicious and nourishing dressing for fruit salads.

BUTTERMILK DRESSING

¾ cup buttermilk
1 egg, well-beaten
1 tbsp. sunflower or sesame seed meal
2½ tsp. butter

2 tsp. lemon juice or wine vinegar
2 scant tsp. honey or raw sugar
½ tsp. salt
⅛ tsp. dry mustard (optional)

Mix together the meal, salt and mustard (if used) in the top of a double boiler. Moisten with about 2 tablespoons of the buttermilk, then stir in the balance of the buttermilk, honey or sugar and well-beaten egg. Place over the bottom of the double boiler in which the water is boiling rapidly. Cook until the dressing thickens, stirring constantly. Remove from the fire, and add the lemon juice or vinegar and the butter. Allow to cool, then chill in the refrigerator before using. This is an inexpensive dressing that is delicious on cole slaw and all the fresh or cooked vegetable salads.

LOW-CALORIE SALAD DRESSING

½ cup dry cottage cheese
½ cup tomato juice

1 clove garlic
pinch of salt
1 tsp. lemon juice

Beat the tomato juice (in which the split garlic clove has steeped for several hours) into the cottage cheese about 1 teaspoon at a time, adding the salt and lemon juice last. Chill and serve with seafood salads, tossed salads or plain vegetable salad; in fact, with all salads except fruit. For a low-calorie fruit salad dressing, omit the garlic and substitute ½ cup orange juice and ¼ teaspoon honey for the tomato juice.

HUNGARIAN YOGURT DRESSING

1 cup yogurt
1 tsp. lemon juice

2 tbsp. chopped chives or green onions

½ tsp. celery salt
4 tbsp. chopped green or ripe olives

1 tbsp. chili sauce or tomato ketchup
1 finely chopped hard-cooked egg

Beat the lemon juice into the yogurt, add the other ingredients and blend well. Chill before serving. This salad dressing contains a definite protein value. Try it on seafood, egg and vegetable salads for its distinctive flavoring.

SWEET BASIL DRESSING

½ cup salad oil (olive, peanut, corn or sunflower)
3 tbsp. lemon juice or wine vinegar

3 tbsp. chopped fresh, or crumbled dried, sweet basil leaves
1 clove garlic
salt to taste

Whip the lemon juice, sweet basil and salt into the oil, drop in the clove of garlic and place in a bottle or jar with an opening for easy pouring. Keep this dressing in a cool dark place, but do *not* place in the refrigerator, as the oil will partially solidify if allowed to become too cold. This makes a wonderful dressing for vegetable, egg and fish salads. Omit the sweet basil and substitute 5 tbsp. of crumbled Gorgonzola, Roquefort or Bleu cheese for a dressing that is unbeatable on tossed green salads. But make certain to stir the dressing well before using, since the cheese will settle to the bottom.

Chapter 28

DELICIOUS BAKING WITH PROTEIN FOODS

No BREAD merits a place in your Eat-and-Grow-Younger menus unless it is truly protein. And only the 100 per cent whole-grain breads can be protein. The breads, rolls, pancakes and waffles made with the recipes given in this chapter may be eaten with the assurance that they do not violate any rules of good nutrition, as do the white-flour and white-sugar products of the oven and griddle; and with the knowledge that these whole-grain breads are contributing valuable proteins, minerals and vitamins to your youth-protecting diet.

You will want to use discretion and balance, of course, in the use of breads the same as with any other food. Don't make a meal of nothing but bread and coffee, for example. Or don't stuff yourself on waffles to the exclusion of meats, eggs, cheese, milk, vegetables and fruits. The only proper way to incorporate breads into the Basic High-Protein Menu is by utilizing their protein contribution to augment your total daily quota of protein grams.

The same is true of cakes, pies and cookies. These foods, as commonly prepared, have no place in any diet because the devitalized all-starch white flour and white sugar from which they are made contain no protein, vitamins or minerals. In other words, to eat such highly artificial baked foods is merely to load up the stomach with something that contributes no nutritive elements, and only slows down the digestive processing of other natural foods.

Yet a nourishing cake, pie or batch of cookies can be made with flours and sweeteners that have genuine food value—and without sacrificing one iota of their deliciousness.

In fact, you've never tasted really wonderful pie until you've eaten one made with a crust of whole-grain flour. And the delicacy and full flavor of a sponge cake or a cheese cake made with whole-grain flour and natural sweeteners can never be equaled by those made with sickly white flour and sugar. You'll quickly discover that confining your consumption of baked foods to those made with whole-grains is no sacrifice—rather, it's a taste privilege.

For making cakes, cookies, waffles and pastry crusts, whole-wheat pastry flour is not necessary, provided the whole-wheat flour is sifted three times, and the coarse husks are removed each time from the sifter. Of course, you don't throw away these coarse particles; you replace them in the flour sack to be used for bread-making. A whole-wheat pastry flour is available in some communities. But if you can't find such a product, don't use that as an excuse for falling back on the old devitalized, all-starch white flour, because the triple sifting will give you cakes and pie crusts just as light-textured as the whole-wheat pastry flour. However, if the whole-wheat pastry flour is available at a health food store near you, then by all means use it for greater convenience.

For breads and rolls you may use your own favorite recipes, substituting for the white flour two-thirds whole-grain flour and one-third millet meal. For muffins, waffles and pancakes, substitute half millet meal and half whole-grain flour. Adding raw wheat germ to all of your baking deserves serious consideration—because it will add so much to nutrition. Replace about 20% of the flour with wheat germ.

Whole-grain flour may be substituted in any recipe calling

for white flour by using approximately *one-fifth more moisture,* and about *10 per cent less shortening.* (The whole-wheat flour absorbs moisture more readily than the devitalized white flour.) For instance, if your recipe calls for 2 cups of white flour, ¾ cup of milk and ½ cup of shortening, all you have to do in order to substitute whole-grain flour for the white flour is this: Increase the milk by one-fifth (since 1 cup equals 16 tablespoons, ¾ cup of milk would be equivalent to 12 tablespoons, and an increase of one-fifth would be approximately 2½ tablespoons more milk). Reduce the shortening by 10 per cent or 1/10 (½ cup shortening would equal 8 tablespoons, and 1/10 less would be 8/10 of a tablespoon, or a very scant tablespoon of shortening).

You may avoid the need for these "kitchen mathematics" by following the basic bread, pancake, waffle, pie, cake and cookie recipes provided below. But each homemaker usually has a favorite recipe which she is loath to give up, so I've given these substitution measurements in order that she may prepare the same old standby baking recipes with whole-grain flours.

From the homemaker's standpoint, another great advantage in whole-grain bread is that it requires *no kneading,* and is therefore much easier to prepare. It's only the pure-starch, devitalized, white-flour breads that require laborious kneading to make them light and palatable.

If you want to increase the protein value of your bread, use all milk, or half milk and half water, and add a beaten egg to the dough. A bread made with egg is also lighter in texture.

BASIC WHOLE-GRAIN BREAD (1 loaf)

3½ cups whole-wheat flour	2 tsp. salt
2 tbsp. powdered skim milk	dash of nutmeg
¾ cup cold water	1 cake compressed yeast, or
¾ cup milk	1 pkg. dry powdered yeast
4 tbsp. honey or raw sugar	¼ cup lukewarm water
2 tbsp. butter or cooking oil	

Dissolve the yeast in the ¼ cup lukewarm water (be sure it is no more than lukewarm, otherwise you'll kill your yeast) together with sugar or honey, until the mixture looks foamy. Scald the ¾ cup of milk with the ¾ cup of cold water, adding the shortening and salt, then cook to lukewarm. Make sure that the flour is room temperature before using, because cold flour will retard the action of the yeast. Sift the nutmeg and the powdered milk with the flour. Add the dissolved yeast and sugar to the liquid milk-and-shortening mixture, then stir thoroughly into the flour, using a wooden batter spoon. If the dough appears too stiff, add enough more lukewarm water to make a stiff, yet soft, dough. Then place the mixing bowl in a large pan (a dishpan is ideal) of very warm water, although not boiling. Cover the bowl with a heavy pastry cloth or tea towel, and allow the dough to rise, which usually takes from 1½ to 2 hours. If the dough is too stiff it won't rise as it should, so you will have to add a tiny bit of lukewarm water to soften up the dough. Before removing from the bowl into a well-greased, large-size bread pan, stir the dough vigorously with the wooden spoon for about 1 minute. Then place the dough in the bread pan, patting into loaf shape with the spoon, cover, and allow to rise again in a warm place protected from drafts (the oven is a good place) for about 45 minutes to 1 hour, or until it almost doubles its bulk. Bake in a moderate oven (350° F.) for about 45 to 50 minutes. If the bread seems to be browning too quickly, turn the oven down. When through baking, immediately turn the loaf out of the pan onto a breadboard or cooling rack, grease the top crust well with either butter or cooking oil (corn or peanut oil is fine for this purpose), then turn the loaf onto its side to cool, covering with a thin cloth. You'll never want to eat "store-bought" bread again once you've tasted this wonderfully delicious, full-flavored bread.

Variations: Use one-third millet meal and two-thirds whole-wheat flour, and increase the sugar or honey to 4½ tablespoons. For raisin bread, add ½ cup of raisins to the flour before adding the liquid. A further addition of sliced citron and orange peel makes a delicious fruit bread that is as good as cake, and which is doubly appreciated in lunch boxes. For extra nutrition, add ¼ cup of raw wheat germ to the flour before mixing in the liquid. This bread may be made without the 2 tablespoons of powdered skim milk, but adding it gives the bread that much extra protein and calcium.

SUNSHINE BREAD (1 loaf)

1¾ cups sunflower seed meal	1¼ cups boiling water
1¾ cups whole-wheat flour	⅓ cup lukewarm water
⅓ cup raisins	1 cake compressed yeast, or
2 tbsp. cooking oil or butter	1 pkg. dry powdered yeast
2 tsp. salt	dash of nutmeg, mace or cin-
4 tbsp. honey or raw sugar	namon

Dissolve the yeast in the lukewarm water, together with the honey or sugar until the mixture looks foamy. Allow the water, to which has been added the fat and salt, to boil, then cool to lukewarm. Sift the sunflower seed meal, flour and spice together, then add the raisins, mixing well. Combine the yeast with the lukewarm water and shortening, then beat thoroughly into the flour. The dough must be well-beaten, yielding a sponge that is soft, yet with some bulk to it. Set to rise as instructed in the previous recipe, and proceed as with Basic Whole-Grain Bread. Remove from pan at once, and treat as instructed in the previous recipe.

TASTY TOAST BREAD (2 loaves)

2⅓ cups whole-wheat flour	1 cup water
1⅔ cups buckwheat flour	1 cup liquid milk made extra
⅓ cup millet meal or sun- flower seed meal	protein-rich by adding 2 tbsp. powdered skim milk
4 tbsp. honey or raw sugar	½ cup lukewarm water
3 tbsp. butter or cooking oil	1 cake compressed yeast, or
2 tsp. salt	1 pkg. of powdered yeast

This bread makes the best toast you ever ate, and it's full of nourishment. Dissolve the yeast, together with 1 tablespoon of the sugar or honey in the ½ cup of lukewarm water. Scald the milk and 1 cup water together, then add the remainder of the sugar or honey, salt and shortening. When cooled to luke-warm, mix in the yeast, and beat thoroughly into the three flours which have been sifted together. Beat well for several minutes. If the dough seems too stiff add a little more luke-warm water; or, if too thin, a little more whole-wheat flour. Proceed as directed in the Basic Whole-Grain Bread recipe given above. Bake in a moderate oven (350° F.) for about 40 to 50 minutes.

SUNFLOWER ORANGE BREAD

¼ cup sunflower seed kernels	2 tsp. baking powder
½ cup pitted, chopped dates juice and rind of 1 large orange	⅓ cup, plus 3 tbsp. raw sugar
2 tbsp. butter or cooking oil	1 well-beaten egg
2½ cups whole-wheat flour	enough milk to make a fairly stiff batter

Add the orange juice and melted shortening to the well-beaten egg, and stir into the sifted ingredients which have been combined with the sugar, chopped dates, orange rind and chopped sunflower seed kernels. Then add enough milk (not too cold) to make a slightly stiffened pouring batter, equivalent to the thickness of the average cake batter. Pour into a well-greased loaf or tube pan, sprinkle the top generously with sunflower seed kernels and bake in a moderate oven (350° F.) for about 1 to 1½ hours (less time if a tube pan is used, of course).

SUNSHINE MUFFINS

½ cup sunflower seed meal
1¼ cups whole-wheat flour
3 tsp. baking powder
¾ tsp. salt
¾ cup milk

3 tbsp. melted butter or cooking oil
3 tbsp. raw sugar or honey
1 large egg

Sift the dry ingredients together. Beat the egg well and stir in the milk (honey also, if used instead of sugar) and melted shortening. Combine with the sifted dry ingredients, stirring only enough to hold the ingredients together. Muffin batter should not even be smooth. Overbeating causes "tunnels" and an uneven grain, and toughens the muffin. Bake in a 9-muffin tin that has been well-greased and floured, for 12 to 15 minutes in a hot oven (400° F.) Remove the pan from the oven as soon as done, and serve at once with butter. Be sure to fill the pans only about one-third full. For variety, add 3 tablespoons of plumped raisins. Any leftover muffins may be split and toasted under the broiler for a teatime snack.

WHOLE-GRAIN WAFFLES

1½ cups whole-wheat flour
½ cup millet meal
2 tbsp. powdered skim milk
½ tsp. salt
1 tbsp. raw sugar or honey

1¾ cups milk
8 tbsp. cooking oil or melted butter
2 eggs, separated and well-beaten

Sift together the dry ingredients, including the milk powder. Add the liquid milk and sweetening to the well-beaten egg yolks and mix with the dry ingredients. Stir in the melted shortening, and fold in last the stiffly beaten egg whites. Bake on a preheated waffle griddle. If you like your waffles good and crisp, here's the trick: Don't close the waffle iron until the batter stops bubbling. This allows the steam to escape and makes a much crisper waffle than if the iron is closed immediately after pouring in the batter. For variety and extra food value, add 3 tablespoons of raw wheat germ to the batter before folding in the egg whites. Chopped pecans or sunflower seed kernels may also be added for delicious nut waffles. As a variation in the syrups to serve with pancakes and waffles, try mixing ⅔ cup honey with an equal amount of heavy sweet or sour cream. This is equally good on cereals. Or melt ⅔ cup of honey in ⅔ cup of hot orange juice with 3 tablespoons of butter, and 1 tablespoon of lemon juice.

NECTAR SPONGE CAKE

6 eggs, separated	2 tsp. lemon juice
1½ cups whole-wheat flour	2 tsp. grated lemon rind
1 tsp. baking powder	½ tsp. salt
1 cup honey	

Separate the eggs, being careful not to get any of the yolk in the whites or they won't beat stiffly enough. Add the salt to the egg whites and beat until they are stiff and stand in little peaks, but are still glossy and not dry. Add the lemon juice and grated rind to the egg yolks and beat until they are thick and lemon-colored. Use a rotary egg beater. Bring the honey to a boil and slowly pour into the egg whites, beating constantly. Fold the egg yolk mixture into the egg whites, then sift the flour (which previously has been sifted three times with the baking powder) over the egg mixture about ¼ cup at a time, and fold carefully, and thoroughly, into the batter before sifting in another ¼ cup of flour, repeating until all the flour is blended into the dough. Do not beat a sponge cake batter, otherwise you will beat the air out of the whites. Place in an *ungreased* tube pan (an angel food cake pan is ideal) and bake in a moderately slow (325° F.) oven for about 1 hour. Turn the cake pan upside down on a cooling rack so the cake will loosen from the sides of the pan as it cools and gradually drop out. Serve plain, with crushed fruits and whipped cream, or with fruits and a custard sauce. This non-fat cake is allowable in small portions on a reducing diet.

SESAME SEED COOKIES

¼ cup whole-wheat flour	1 egg, well-beaten
½ cup raw sugar	pinch of salt
½ tsp. baking powder	½ tsp. vanilla or almond extract
¼ cup (4 tbsp.) butter or cooking oil	½ cup sesame seeds

Cream the shortening and sugar together until very fluffy, then add 1 tablespoon of the sifted dry ingredients before mixing in the well-beaten egg, flavoring and sesame seeds (these may previously be browned slightly in the oven if desired) before blending in thoroughly the remainder of the flour which may or may not be triple-sifted, according to your taste. (For a thicker, softer cookie use ⅓ cup of flour.) Drop by small spoonfuls, widely spaced, onto a greased and floured baking sheet or cookie pan. Bake about 8 minutes at 375° F. The recipe as given yields a thin, crisp wafer.

SESAME DATE BARS

1 cup dates, chopped
1 cup sesame seeds, browned (chopped sunflower seed kernels may be used instead)

1 tsp. baking powder
4 tsp. whole-wheat flour
¾ cup raw sugar
2 eggs, well-beaten
¼ tsp. vanilla

Beat the eggs very well, then add the sugar, and continue beating. Stir in the dates and sesame seeds, blending in last the flour well-mixed with the baking powder. Spread the dough in a shallow greased pan. Bake in a very slow oven (250° to 275° F.) for about 15 to 20 minutes. While still hot, cut into small bars or squares. These cookies are almost a "candy bar," because they contain so little flour, yet the sesame seeds and eggs give them a high-protein content.

GRANDMOTHER'S MOLASSES COOKIES

½ cup butter
1 cup raw sugar
1 cup thick sour cream or yogurt
2 eggs, well beaten
1 cup molasses (dark sorghum or pure cane, and for a different flavor try maple syrup)

4½ cups whole-wheat flour
2 tsp. soda
¼ tsp. nutmeg
¼ tsp. cinnamon
⅛ tsp. cloves
   dash of ginger

Cream the sugar and shortening until fluffy, then gradually beat in the molasses, 2 tablespoons of the sifted dry ingredients (except the soda), and the well-beaten eggs. Mix the soda with the yogurt or sour cream, and add gradually, alternating with the sifted dry ingredients. Chill in the refrigerator for several hours, then drop by the tablespoonful onto a well-oiled cookie sheet or shallow rectangular pan. Bake in a moderate oven (350° F.) for about 12 minutes. This recipe makes about 6 to 7 dozen of the kind of molasses cookie that grown men dream about having eaten at "grandmother's house."

SOUR CREAM PIE CRUST

½ cup sour cream (ice cold)
¼ tsp. soda
3 tbsp. soft butter
¼ tsp. salt
½ tsp. almond extract
1¼ cups whole-wheat flour, triple-sifted (chilled in the refrigerator)

Sift the flour (already triple-sifted) with the salt and soda into a large bowl. Add the almond extract to the sour cream, then gradually mix into the flour to form a soft dough. Divide the dough in half. Knead one portion slightly on a floured board or pastry cloth, and roll out to fit a pie tin. Place in the refrigerator. Roll out the remainder of the dough and spread with the soft butter. Fold over and roll out several times more in order to work the butter into the dough. Roll out again on a pastry cloth, and chill thoroughly in the refrigerator for use as the flaky top crust (the extra butter makes it flaky). Meanwhile prepare the pie filling and place in the pan with the bottom crust. Cover with the chilled top crust and bake in a hot oven. This is an excellent basic pie crust recipe for any kind of pie. For an open-faced pie, use half the recipe, or else make the entire recipe, saving half the dough in the refrigerator for the next day. You'll note that I use almond extract in my pie crusts. This is a trick I learned from the Italian master chef in one of the swankiest hotels in Montevideo.

WHOLE-GRAIN CHEESE CRUST

1 cup whole-wheat flour, triple-sifted
1 tsp. salt
⅓ cup ice-cold shortening (cooking oil or butter)
½ cup grated snappy cheese
2 tbsp. shortening at room temperature
ice water

Sift the flour (already triple-sifted) with the salt. Add the grated cheese. Cut into the ice-cold shortening with a pastry blender or two knives until evenly mixed and of the consistency of coarse sand. Add the ice water a few drops at a time, stirring lightly with a fork, using only enough water to make the particles of flour-and-fat hold together. It's not important that the dough hold together in one firm ball, just enough so it may be lifted out onto a floured board or pastry canvas. Roll out thick (with a minimum of handling) and spread with the warm shortening, fold double, and then roll out again to about ⅛-inch thickness. This is an excellent crust for a whole-wheat apple pie, for meat and vegetable pies, for cheese straws, or cheese wafers to be eaten with soup, or for snacks. For a two-crust pie, double the recipe.

SUNSHINE NUT TORTE

2 eggs, well-beaten
2 cups milk
¼ cup chopped sunflower seed kernels
2½ tbsp. honey
¼ cup chopped pistachio nuts (hazelnuts, blanched almonds or pecans may be used instead)

1 tbsp. browned sesame seeds (optional)
¾ cup whole-wheat flour, triple-sifted
¼ tsp. nutmeg
⅛ tsp. almond extract
pinch of salt
1 recipe Torte Egg Crust (see page 215)

Use a deep saucepan, or top of a double boiler, and gradually blend the milk into the flour until the mixture is smooth. Then add the honey, well-beaten eggs, nutmeg and salt. Beat until thoroughly blended. Place over a low flame, or over boiling water, and bring to a boil, stirring constantly to prevent lumping and sticking. Gradually stir in the sunflower and nut kernels chopped medium-fine, until the mixture is smooth custard. Remove from the fire and cool, then stir in the almond extract. When cool pour into a pie plate lined with Torte Egg Crust, and place crisscross strips over the top, pinching the edges of the strips into the edge of the bottom crust. Bake in a moderately hot oven (350° to 375° F.) for about 45 minutes, or until the custard is firm, and the crust a nice golden brown. Remove from the oven and cool before serving.

SOUR CREAM FRUIT PIE

½ cup raw sugar, or honey
1 tbsp. whole-wheat flour
1 cup sour cream (or yogurt)

3 cups fruit or berries (fresh or canned)
1 recipe Sour Cream Pie Crust

Combine the sugar and flour. If honey is used, blend it into the sour cream, then add to the flour. Line a 10-inch pie pan with half the dough, as directed in the recipe for Sour Cream Pie Crust. Fill with well-washed and drained fresh fruits or berries, or with drained canned fruit. Pour the cream and flour mixture over them, blending in well so all the fruit is coated with cream. If a top crust is used, it may be placed solid or in lattice strips ½-inch wide. Bake for 10 minutes at 450 F., then lower to 325° and continue baking for about 30 minutes longer. If the bottom crust is first coated with unbeaten egg white before filling with the fruit, it will remain drier and not soak up the fruit juices.

OLD-TIME BUTTERMILK CUSTARD PIE

3 eggs, separated	1 tbsp. lemon juice
1 cup raw sugar	2 tbsp. orange juice
3 tbsp. whole-wheat flour	1 tsp. each of grated lemon
2 cups buttermilk	and orange rind
¼ tsp. salt	½ recipe for Sour Cream
4 tbsp. butter	Pie Crust

Cream the sugar and butter together, and stir in the flour, salt, fruit juices and grated rind. Add the well-beaten egg yolks mixed with the buttermilk. Beat until smooth. Fold in last the stiffly beaten egg whites. Pour the custard mixture into a 10-inch pie pan lined with half the recipe for Sour Cream Pie Crust. Bake for 10 minutes at 450° F., then reduce to 350° and continue baking for 30 to 35 minutes longer, or until the custard is firmly set in the center when tested with a knife blade. Whenever you serve this old-time custard pie, you may be certain it adds valuable nutrients to your daily diet.

COTTAGE CHEESE PINEAPPLE PIE

1 cup cottage cheese	2 tbsp. lemon juice
½ cup drained, crushed pine-apple	1 cup thin cream
	½ recipe Sour Cream Pie
2 eggs, separated	Crust or Torte Egg Crust
7 tbsp. raw sugar	

Combine the cream, lemon juice and well-beaten egg yolks. Beat into the cottage cheese, then add the pineapple and 3 tablespoons of the sugar, mixing well. Pour into a 9-inch baked pastry shell. Top with a meringue made by beating the egg whites together with a little salt until they stand in peaks, then adding the remainder of the sugar. Brown the meringue in a slow oven (300° F.) for about 20 minutes, taking care not to overcook, or the meringue will become tough and rubbery. Chill before serving. For variety, add about ⅓ cup shredded coconut.

TORTE EGG CRUST

4 tbsp. butter	¼ tsp. salt
½ cup raw sugar	1 egg, lightly beaten
2 cups whole-wheat flour, triple sifted	2 tbsp. cooking sherry or orange juice

Sift the ingredients together (the flour is already triple-sifted). Blend in the butter with a pastry mixer. Add the lightly-beaten egg, and gradually stir in enough cooking sherry or orange juice to make a firm pastry dough. It may take more or less than the specified amount, depending on the flour. For a torte or cream pie, roll out a circular piece of dough about ⅛-inch thick to fit a 9- or 10-inch pie pan. Grease the pan before fitting in the crust. Pinch the edges to make an even fluted upstanding rim. Then cut the remainder of the dough into strips ½-inch wide to make a crisscross lattice top crust.

Chapter 29

SWEETS AND TREATS THAT ARE "DIVIDENDS"

DESSERTS certainly provide a pleasant way of topping off a meal. And a sweet or delicious beverage once in a while is a mouth-watering treat to anticipate. Most assuredly I have no intention of denying you these taste pleasures in your Eat-and-Grow-Younger diet.

What I am suggesting is that you limit your desserts, sweets and between-meal beverages to those that "carry their own weight" in your youth-protecting diet. In other words, to desserts, sweets and treat beverages that are *dividends*—that add extra protein, minerals and vitamins to your daily intake of nutrients.

How can you determine which sweets to discard?

Easy enough—by their over-all content of vital food elements. How much protein, for instance, is there in a slice of white-flour cake frosted with white-sugar icing; how many minerals in a piece of chocolate candy; how many vitamins in a white-flour crusted pie filled with a ready-mix artificially flavored and colored "pudding"? For all practical purposes, the answer is "absolutely none"!

That is what I mean by insisting that a dessert, sweet or treat beverage should carry its own weight. Eggs, milk, yogurt, cottage cheese, nuts, seeds, fruits, honey, raw sugar—these foods all possess something of nutritional worth to contribute to your diet program, and I have used them in numerous different combinations in all the foregoing recipes. We shall now re-combine all these highly nutritious foods into other delicious forms in order to produce desserts, sweets and beverages that are a genuine nutritive addition to any diet.

However, I don't mean to imply by this that you may overindulge in these taste treats to the neglect of meat and vegetable dishes at mealtime. A dividend means exactly what it implies—*a small extra portion given as a compensation.*

In this instance, the desserts, sweets and beverages given below are allowed you as a "compensation" for abandoning the health-wrecking artificial cakes, candies, pastries and soft drinks that add nothing to your diet except coal-tar dyes and flavorings, and youth-destroying starches.

ORANGE CHIFFON

3 egg yolks	1 tbsp. gelatin, unflavored
2½ tbsp. honey or raw sugar	juice of 4 oranges
1 cup thin cream	grated rind of 1 orange
1 cup whipping cream	grated rind of ½ lemon

Beat the egg yolks slightly in the top of a double boiler, then stir in the sugar (or honey), thin cream and grated citrus peel. Place over boiling water and beat with a rotary egg beater until the mixture thickens, taking care not to let it boil. Remove from the fire, and add the gelatin which has been dissolved in ¼ cup of cold water 5 minutes previously. Stir well, then pour into a deep bowl and continue beating until partially cool. Beat in the orange juice, then fold in the whipped cream. Pour into a mold that has been well rinsed in cold water, and place in in the refrigerator to set. This makes about 6 servings. Instead of commercial ice cream, made with white sugar, artificial flavorings and colorings and thickening powders, prepare this chiffon cream for dessert or party refreshments. It's as good nutrition as it is good eating.

MILK PUDDING

2½ cups milk
2 tbsp. butter
3 tbsp. honey or raw sugar
5 tbsp. millet meal
1 tbsp. sesame seed or sunflower seed meal
1 tsp. grated lemon rind

3 eggs, separated (if small, use 4)
¾ cup cooked apples, apricots, or crushed pineapple
¼ cup shredded coconut (optional)

Melt the butter in a heavy saucepan. Add the sugar, or honey, and 2 cups of the milk (reserving ½ cup to be mixed into a paste with the flour), and let come to a boil. Stir in the flour-milk paste and cook for 4 to 5 minutes longer. Remove from the fire and pour into a bowl to cool. Then stir in the beaten egg yolks into which have been mixed the grated lemon peel and the seed meal. Cut in the stiffly beaten whites with a silver knife. Pour the mixture into a well-greased baking dish and bake in a moderate oven until the pudding is about half done. Remove from the oven, and spread the cooked fruit quickly over the top, then sprinkle with the coconut if used. Return to the oven as quickly as possible to finish baking. Serve while hot. This makes about 6 portions.

DUCHESS CREAM PUDDING

2 cups milk
1 cup powdered skim milk
3 tbsp. raw sugar or honey

1½ tsp. vanilla
1 junket tablet
1 tbsp. water

Beat the milk powder into the liquid milk with a rotary egg beater. Add the sugar or honey and beat until smooth. Heat the milk to lukewarm (110° F. on a candy thermometer), but *do not overheat*. Remove from fire and add the junket tablet which has been dissolved in the 1 tablespoon of cold water. Blend well into the warmed milk together with the vanilla. Pour at once into individual serving dishes (about 4 portions) and allow to stand in a warm room until set. Then chill. Serve with crushed fresh or canned fruit, berries or orange slices. Whipped cream may be used as a topping. Pure vegetable colorings (be sure to read your labels when buying food colorings, for most of them are coal-tar, aniline dyes) may be used to tint this delicious junket pudding for extra eye appeal. The added powdered milk makes this an extremely high-protein dessert, although a light, easily digested one, and a far creamier junket pudding than the ordinary kind. Serve this high-protein pudding with a meatless meal, or one whose quota of protein grams is below normal. Because of its low-calorie count, this makes a splendid dessert for the reducing diet.

LEMON MILK SHERBET

3 cups milk	6 tbsp. honey
3 tbsp. grated lemon rind	½ cup raw sugar
¾ cup lemon juice	3 eggs

Beat the eggs until slightly thickened, add the sugar and continue beating. Stir in the honey, lemon juice and grated rind, blending the milk in gradually at the last. Pour into the refrigerator tray and freeze at highest speed. When mushy, remove from the refrigerator, stir vigorously or whip the sherbet to break up the ice crystals, then continue freezing. This sherbet is usually a "man's favorite." Serve it with a meat meal for a light, yet nourishing, dessert. Or keep some in the refrigerator (in the deep freeze, too) for a family or party treat. This recipe makes a little more than 1 quart.

BAVARIAN FRUIT WHIP

1 cup whipping cream	⅓ cup chopped nuts
1 cup mixed fresh, canned, or frozen fruit (pineapple, peaches, bananas, strawberries, raspberries, blueberries, sweet cherries)	1 tbsp. honey
	1 tsp. vanilla

Whip the cream, and add the vanilla and honey. Mix well with the fruit and chill. Serve in sherbet glasses, and garnish the top with a candied cherry and two green citron slices. This is a light, easily prepared dessert that is fancy enough to serve for "company" meals.

APRICOT DAINTIES

¾ cup dried apricots	1 tsp. each grated orange and lemon peel
½ cup nut meats	
¾ cup coconut	1 tbsp. lemon juice
2 tbsp. powdered skim milk	

Put the apricots, nuts and coconut through the food chopper. Add the grated citrus peel and the milk powder, blending thoroughly. Moisten with the lemon juice. If desired, roll in ground toasted coconut or nuts. This makes approximately 50 small balls; or the mixture may be shaped into rolls, thoroughly chilled and sliced; or packed into a loaf pan and cut into squares. Pack several pieces of this health sweet into lunches for the morning and afternoon pick-up desired by the school child or working person. How much safer from a health standpoint to nibble on this protein-containing natural sweet than to insult the stomach with candy bars or soft drinks.

SESAME SEED BALLS

½ cup sesame seeds
2 tbsp. honey
½ lb. dried apricots

1 lb. pitted dates
⅓ cup seedless raisins

Brown the sesame seeds slightly in the oven. Run all the fruit through the food chopper. Add the honey and blend thoroughly. Shape into small balls and roll in the browned sesame seeds, adding more honey if necessary to coat each piece well. If you were to travel in the Grecian isles of the Mediterranean, you'd very likely be served this delicious sesame seed confection.

SESAME SEED BUTTER CREAMS

½ cup browned sesame seeds
1 cup milk
½ cup butter

¾ cup raw sugar, plus another ¼ cup
few drops vanilla

Boil the ¾ cup of sugar, butter and milk together until the mixture barely forms a soft ball in cold water. Meanwhile caramelize* the remaining ¼ cup of sugar in a heavy iron skillet so that the two are ready at the same time. Quickly scrape the caramelized syrup into the milk mixture, beating until it becomes quite thick, then add the seeds which previously have been lightly browned in the oven, and the vanilla. If the mixture seems slow in thickening, set in a pan of cold water. Drop by the teaspoonful onto a buttered platter to harden. When cold, this recipe makes about 2 dozen pieces of creamy candy with a real protein value, owing to its sesame seeds and milk.

* The process of melting and browning sugar in a skillet until light brown and having a caramel flavor.

SESAME SEED TAFFY TWISTS

⅓ cup browned sesame seeds   1 tbsp. butter
⅓ cup cream   1⅓ cup brown or raw sugar
⅓ cup molasses   a few drops vanilla

Boil the cream, sugar, molasses and butter to the stage where a little dropped into cold water forms a harder-than-soft-ball (about 240° to 244° F. on a candy thermometer). Add the sesame seeds and vanilla and beat until the mixture becomes quite thick. Drop by small spoonfuls onto a greased cookie sheet or platter, then chill in the refrigerator. When cool the candy is still slightly soft, and may be rolled into little balls or patties, and wrapped in twists of waxed paper. If kept chilled in the refrigerator until eaten, the candy will not stick to the paper.

There you have it—some basic recipe ideas from which you will make your own variations and adaptations as you follow the Eat-and-Grow-Younger program.

Good luck to you—all the way!

TO MY READERS

In the years to come I hope to see an even keener interest displayed in health through good nutrition. Nutritional therapy has made great strides . . . it must make still greater advances before the American people can truthfully be considered a healthy, vigorous nation.

The fact that you purchased a copy of this book is proof in itself that you are interested in your body . . . and how to keep it nutritionally healthy. I want to help you as much as I can.

The thousands of health students throughout the world whom it has been my pleasure to address time and time again will find much of my lecture material in this book, amplified by the very latest discoveries in nutritional science. To them this volume is dedicated; their loyalty and enthusiasm have been a real inspiration to me.

Of course, the time will come when the information set forth herein will need to be supplemented by reports of the latest discoveries to come from research laboratories all over the world. And I feel it is my obligation to you, as a reader of my book, that these latest reports come to your attention.

For that reason I publish, from time to time, bulletins on health and nutrition. These are sent, FREE OF ANY COST, *to all who are interested in my work. If you would like to receive these reports as they are issued, kindly drop me a postal card and your name will be placed on our mailing list. (You will of course be automatically notified when I am scheduled to lecture in your city.)*

LELORD KORDEL

Box 4834 Redford Station
Detroit 19, Michigan

SEXUAL VIGOR AND NUTRITION

The book that lets women know what men want in women, both in and out of bed, and tells you how you can become a more desirable woman for the man in your life. And all it takes is a better diet. Poor nutrition can ruin your looks, bring your spirits down and take away from your sex appeal. Don't let that happen. This book can improve the total you.

15181—$1.50

HEALTH THROUGH NUTRITION

Avoid costly visits to the doctor and high-priced medications. Costly problems such as arthritis, insomnia, fatigue, indigestion, neurosis, high blood pressure and heart disease can often be avoided— easily and inexpensively. Even your I.Q. can be elevated. The world-famous nutritionist, Lelord Kordel tells you how. Eating the right foods, getting the correct nutrition can help you feel healthier, live longer and enjoy life to its fullest.

17121—$1.75

EAT & GROW YOUNGER

All you need to feel and look younger is a better diet. Avoid expensive face-lifts, plastic surgery, doctor visits and drugs. They are only temporary solutions to the problems of aging. They attack the problem after the damage is done, and they don't help you feel younger, either physically or mentally. All you really need is a simple, well-balanced diet, with less sugar and more protein. Lelord Kordel, the world-renowned nutritionist, devised an easy-to-follow routine which will lessen the effects of aging. This book can help you to attain a more youthful body and mind. You can learn to enjoy life to the fullest and always feel your best.

#15186—$1.50

Manor Books, Inc.
432 Park Avenue South
New York, New York 10016

Please send me the books I have checked above. I am enclosing $_____ Check or money order, (no currency or C.O.D.'s). Enclose price listed for each title plus 25¢ per copy ordered to cover cost of postage and handling.

Send me a free list of all your books in print.

Name _____

Address _____

City _____ State _____ Zip _____